The Spiritual Challenge of Health Care

For Churchill Livingstone:

Senior Commissioning Editor: Alex Mathieson
Project Manager: Valerie Burgess
Project Development Editor: Valerie Dearing
Copy Editor: Colin Macnee
Indexer: Tarrant Ranger Indexing Agency
Design Direction: Judith Wright
Promotions Manager: Hilary Brown

The Spiritual Challenge of Health Care

Edited by

Mark Cobb BSc
Senior Chaplain, Central Sheffield University Hospitals, Sheffield, UK

Vanessa Robshaw BSc PGDip RN
Sister, Department of Genito-Urinary Medicine, Derbyshire Royal Infirmary, Derby, UK

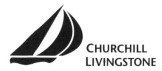

CHURCHILL
LIVINGSTONE

EDINBURGH LONDON NEW YORK PHILADELPHIA SYDNEY TORONTO AND TOKYO 1998

CHURCHILL LIVINGSTONE
An imprint of Harcourt Brace and Company Limited

© Harcourt Brace and Company Limited 1998
© Spiritual care, health care: what's the difference? – Julia Neuberger
© The re-enchantment of health care: a paradigm of spirituality – Pamela Reed

logo is a registered trademark of Harcourt Brace and Company Limited 1998

First published 1998

ISBN 0443 059209

British Library of Cataloguing in Publication Data
A catalogue record for this book is available from the British Library.

Library of Congress Cataloging in Publication Data
A catalog record for this book is available from the Library of Congress.

The
publisher's
policy is to use
**paper manufactured
from sustainable forests**

Produced by Addison Wesley Longman China Limited, Hong Kong
SWTC/01

Contents

Contributors

Editors

Mark Cobb and **Vanessa Robshaw** organised the first national conference on spiritual care, *Body and Soul*, in 1996. They are both involved in training health care professionals and have established a research project on spiritual care in the acute hospital setting. Mark Cobb is the Senior Chaplain of Central Sheffield University Hospitals and was formerly Palliative Care and Health Care Chaplain at the Derbyshire Royal Infirmary. Vanessa Robshaw was formerly a practice and research nurse. She is now a sister in the department of genito-urinary medicine at the Derbyshire Royal Infirmary.

Contributors

Janet Bellamy, BA BLitt MEd PGCE, is a BAC accredited counsellor, a counselling supervisor and a lecturer in counselling at Westhill College of Higher Education in Birmingham. Her previous experience includes teaching and hospital chaplaincy.

Grace Davie, BA PhD, is a senior lecturer in sociology at the University of Exeter and is the convenor of the International Society for the Sociology of Religion. She is the author of *Religion in Britain since 1945*.

Michael D Jacobs, MA(Oxon) FBAC, is a registered psychotherapist, supervisor and a senior lecturer in the Department of Adult Education at the University of Leicester. He is the author and editor of numerous books on pastoral care and counselling, including *Living Illusions*.

Anne Johnson, RGN DipNur, is an experienced registered nurse. She teaches on various aspects of nursing, is an advisor on training needs, and is a senior nurse in Professional Development at the Derbyshire Royal Infirmary.

Ian Markham, BD PhD MLitt, is Holder of the Liverpool Chair of Theology and Public Life at Liverpool Hope University College. He is the author of *A World Religions Reader*.

Julia Neuberger, MA(Cantab), is a Rabbi who is well known for her involvement with health care. She is the Chief Executive Officer of the King's Fund in London and has published many books, including *Caring For Dying People Of Different Faiths.*

Linda A Ross, BA(Nur) PhD RGN, is a registered nurse and former Research Fellow in the Department of Nursing Studies at the University of Edinburgh. She received her doctorate for research into the spiritual aspects of nursing.

Neil Small, BSc PhD MSW, is a Senior Research Fellow at the Trent Palliative Care Centre in Sheffield, and also at the University of Sheffield. His current research interests include the history of the modern hospice movement. His past work has concentrated on people living with AIDS and on the politics of the NHS. He is the author of *AIDS: The Challenge.*

Pamela G Reed is Professor and Associate Dean for Academic Affairs at the Health Sciences Centre of the University of Arizona, teaching metatheory and the philosophy of science. She has researched and published in the fields of spirituality, mental helath and ageing, and works from a developmental perspective.

Peter W Speck, MA BSc, is the chaplaincy team leader for the Southampton University Hospitals and was formerly chaplain and honorary lecturer at the Royal Free Hospital and Medical School in London. He has contributed the only chapter on spiritual care in *The Oxford Textbook of Palliative Medicine.*

Margaret Whipp, BA MBChB MRCP FRCR, is a priest and a consultant clinical oncologist at Weston Park Hospital in Sheffield. She is also Vocations Advisor for the Diocese of Sheffield and has become well known for her work in bridging the gap between science and spirituality.

Preface

The spiritual dimension of health care, whilst frequently recognised as important, is often based upon intuition and a conventional religious approach. The lack of a clear conceptual framework, general uncertainty, and limited opportunities in training and professional development, have resulted in a neglect of this important aspect of patient care.

As a response to this, we conceived a national conference to address these issues and to encourage debate and discussion within the NHS. The conference was entitled *Body & Soul* and provided a unique combination of professional research, practice and experience that stimulated an overwhelming interest. We never imagined when we were planning the conference that the BBC World Service, *The Health Service Journal* and a host of other media organisations would be fascinated by what we regarded as such an obvious and yet unexplored subject.

The response to the conference convinced us there was a need for a book on spiritual care that dealt with the complex challenges of spirituality in health care. This book reflects aspects of spiritual care explored at the first conference and a subsequent conference in 1997, as well as drawing upon wider issues concerning health care professionals in this developing field.

The authors of this book represent a considerable breadth of experience and expertise: each chapter offers a distinctive insight into this multifaceted area of health care. Many health care professionals have contributed to the book, but we have also included specialists in the disciplines of sociology, psychology, counselling and theology for the value of their perspectives in complementing and enhancing clinical knowledge and skills.

It can be argued that spirituality is fundamental to humanity and therefore spiritual care should be considered appropriate for all patients. Traditionally, spiritual care has been synonymous with religious care. However, the multicultural and secular shape of contemporary society has encouraged the development of a broader approach that is able to respect the integrity of particular faith communities and is relevant to those outside of them.

Throughout this book common themes emerge:

- The general inability of health care to deal with the spiritual dimension.

- The impact of illness and injury on the spiritual needs of patients.
- The discounting of spiritual beliefs and values within the dominant scientific paradigm.
- The apparent disparity between the care of the whole person and the treatment of the part.
- The implications of a commitment to spiritual care for training, practice and resources.

This book raises many challenging issues that need to be faced by health care practitioners and those concerned with its provision. Since its inception in 1948 the NHS has recognised the necessity of providing for people's spiritual needs and this book sets out an important new agenda for the future of health care.

Many people have contributed directly and indirectly to this book and deserve our thanks, most especially the staff and patients of the Derbyshire Royal Infirmary. The foundations of this book were shaped by a working party into spiritual care that involved Celiene Smythe-Renshaw and Kevin Skippon. The original conference team of Kaye Burnett, Peggy Jones, Jill Straw and Jane Wain provided vital support and encouragement. Finally, our gratitude to Valerie Dearing and Alex Mathieson of Churchill Livingstone for their enthusiasm and expertise.

MC, VR
Derby 1997

Introduction: body and soul?

Mark Cobb
Vanessa Robshaw

Health care is about bodies: bodies that aren't working properly, bodies that have been damaged and bodies that are ailing. To these bodies we dispense medicine, perform surgery and utilize treatments in an attempt to restore health. By dissecting bodies, and through experiments and discoveries, scientists have led the way in explaining the body, in understanding its functions and in predicting its behaviour. Health care is therefore a perfectly rational exercise, but it is motivated by something that is more fundamental than the physical and chemical manipulation of flesh and blood. It is motivated by a desire to relieve suffering through healing.

People experience suffering in and through their bodies but it is seldom a purely physical affair. It is a response of the person both to the corporal trauma of illness and injury and to the life trauma of adversity and tragedy. Physical pathology is therefore one aspect of suffering which is characteristic of a biomedical model of illness. Other models take into account different perspectives of illness such as the psychology of illness or its demographic characteristics. A sociological model, for example, makes a distinction between disease as scientific observation and illness as a personal experience. Helman (1990) therefore asserts that, 'Illness is the subjective response of the patient, and of course those around him, to his being unwell; particularly how he, and they, interpret the origin and significance of this event. ... It not only includes his experience of ill-health, but also the meaning he gives to the experience'.

A narrative of suffering may be informed by a biomedical model of disease and disorder but it rarely provides a complete or satisfying account, because being human is more than physical existence, and suffering is more than biological malfunction. In all this there is what many people recognize as a spiritual quality to life which, in suffering, confronts people with questions and possibilities that reach beyond the immediate dilemmas of physical insult. This 'sparse' view of spirituality has been

1

described by Bragan (1996) as 'the reality of transcendency, in an experiential sense; from the awareness which carries not only a recognition of the immediate and the concrete, but also a sense of the abstract and timeless; the awareness that life cannot be encompassed by rationality but extends into an unknown; and the awareness that certain experiences have a particular quality bringing uplift of spirit'.

Spirituality may seem to be something of a dusty relic from the religious past when mentioned alongside the gleaming modernity of medical treatment, the soul an arcane remnant of a worldview now succeeded by the captivating picture which science presents. However, ignoring spirituality and writing it out of the accounts of health, wellbeing and suffering will not make it disappear. In particular, as the philosopher Gadamer (1996, p. 13) reflects, 'thanks to the knowledge humans have of themselves, the "science" which seeks to perceive everything that becomes accessible to it with its methodological means is confronted in a special way with the theme "human being". Its task of understanding is posed to it as one that is unending, incomplete, continually in view'. The theme 'human being' is of primary importance to health care, and science provides an important means of describing it, but it has little to say of the life and wellbeing that are fundamental to being human, for that is not its task. If we wish health care to take a more comprehensive account of humanity then we will need to give regard to the spirituality of life that seems evident when that same life is challenged and threatened.

It is all too easy in the constraints of a health care setting to collapse a complex picture into a generic category. It is also tempting in a context in which the scientific perspective is dominant to discount anything outside this frame of reference. But, if health care is concerned with human being as much as human life, with suffering as much as disease and injury, with healing as much as cure, then a shallow picture of humanity will not suffice. The concept of holism would seem to offer an obvious supplement to this partial picture. A holistic approach may be defined as the integration of the physical, social, psychological and spiritual aspects of the person. However, this broader perspective may in fact be an amalgamation of discrete parts rather than an appreciation of the whole human being and all that that involves. Gadamer (1996, p. 115) recalls Plato when he says that 'it is impossible to heal the body without knowing something about the soul, indeed without knowing something about the nature of the "whole"'.

Holistic care is most readily associated with palliative and hospice care. It is perhaps not surprising that in the care of people with terminal illness, when physical cure is unobtainable, that the nature of the whole is advocated which encompasses the spiritual aspects of living and dying. Hospice care can look back to the monastic communities who provided care for the sick, poor and dying out of their sense of vocation. However, the modern hospice movement, evolving out of a critique of terminal care, is oriented less by its religious tradition and more by the speciality of palliative medicine which draws upon secular discourses about death. Thus, whilst a spiritual aspect of care is maintained, often through the presence of a chaplain, it is underpinned less by theology and more by the insights of the social sciences and humanistic philosophy.

In contemporary society, spirituality has become a relativized and fragmented concept which has not found a standard definition. Etymologically, one route returns to the notion of an animating or actuating life force, literally the breath of life. Other ideas, from different faith perspectives, invoke a sense of the transcendent, the sacred and the divine. Whatever account is used is imprinted with cultural themes and bears social and historical motifs. Worldviews, philosophies and beliefs are embedded within particular understandings of spirituality such that any attempt at integrating them is likely to result in a bland common denominator devoid of significant distinctions. Spirituality may be expressed in divergent and complex forms, as witnessed in religions, but this is no reason to deal with it either as beyond comprehension or as limited to meaningless stereotypes.

Many patients have no formal attachment to a faith community. In part, this reflects a general decline in religious practice in contemporary society, but it cannot be assumed that people do not have any beliefs or a spiritual dimension to their lives. Despite the prevalence of secular attitudes, spiritual experiences and expressions persist; the sacred and secular are not mutually exclusive. This is reinforced from a psychological perspective in that beliefs and faith are necessary for human development and in making sense of and finding meaning in life. In this way, spirituality serves a common human purpose which may be disoriented or dislocated in the face of illness, suffering and loss. Thus, a health crisis may precipitate a spiritual challenge which may enrich or diminish a person.

Spirituality, as it has been discussed so far, is a term which can have a wide range of interpretations. There is clearly a need for debate as to the meaning of spirituality and its place in health care, and it is constructive that a dialogue is beginning to emerge among health care disciplines which is generating research, the development of useful models and changes in practice. However, caution and conservatism are apparent in this process, resulting not only from the defence of the boundaries of medical orthodoxy but also from a wish to safeguard the vulnerability of those who are ill.

A specific example offers a relevant insight into this debate. The term 'spirituality' is used by New Age movements whose unconventional and largely unregulated therapies have found some accommodation in mainstream health care. New Age spirituality embraces an eclectic range of ideas and philosophies, often of an esoteric nature, many of which appeal to the advancement of the individual in search of enlightenment and fulfilment. There is, therefore, an incoherence in New Age spirituality which is paradoxically contained within common beliefs and values such as the authority of inner wisdom, the oneness of creation and the utopian goal of the New Age. Lyon (1996) has suggested that the New Age 'may be seen as a cultural resource that is mobilized in response to the spiritual vacuum of modern administered, technological societies, but which in many ways offers escape rather than an engagement with or critique of them'. Whatever the place of spirituality in health care and the nature of its claims and practice, it must be open to rigorous critique and be able to bear the scrutiny of other disciplines in seeking recognition, endorsement and incorporation. The practice of spiritual care within health care settings must also be justified by a plausible rationale and governed by an unambiguous ethical code. It is the involvement with those who are ill and suffer that has inspired the engagement with the spiritual challenge of health care evident in this book, rather than use of spirituality as a means of escaping suffering.

Is there a role for spiritual care in health care? It can be argued that the scientific reductionism of much medical care and the persistent dissatisfaction of the human condition have created a gap which spiritual care can usefully fill. Spiritual care in this sense is a reassertion of the human spirit over and against the sterile materialist world and an indication of the limits of contemporary health care. But spirituality is more than a symptom of dissatisfaction, for when people are confronted with life events concerning their very existence, fundamental spiritual issues often emerge. Spiritual care therefore involves a recovery of the patient as a person, upholding his or her beliefs and experiences and addressing matters of meaning and hope.

Religious faith and practice may be a part of spiritual care, but it will fundamentally concern attending the sick in ways that inspire being human and which open a way for the sharing of faith and doubt, suffering and joy. As one person in the service of another, spiritual care is therefore literally therapeutic, and not an attempt to impose, intervene or control.

Among the doctors of ancient Greece the name of Hippocrates has survived in the form of the oath which remains as a standard of professional ethics and a summary of many of the values and beliefs that have shaped medicine. In an attempt at rewriting the oath in a contemporary form the poet David Hart (1997) captures some important principles that resonate with what has been said so far about spiritual care: '... I will excite the sick and the well by the severity of my kindness to a wholeness of purpose. I shall apply my knowledge, curiosity, ignorance and ability to listen. I shall cooperate with wondering practitioners in the art and the sciences, with all who care for people's bodies and souls, so that the whole person in relationship shall be kept in view, their aspirations and their unease'. Here is a reciprocal relationship between the patient and the caregiver that recognizes the interdependence of each and the nature of the whole. In all this there will be ambiguity, humility and uncertainty because there is much about health and suffering which is hidden out of reach and which cannot provide answers to our searching and sometimes desperate questions.

Health care is, if nothing else, practical: it requires organizing, resources and implementation. Spirituality, therefore, needs to be understood, researched, taught and applied to practice. Any response to the spiritual challenge of health care must include these practical implications otherwise it will remain a rhetorical exercise that has little to offer either those who are burdened with disease or those who care for them.

This book seeks to expand and encourage the discussion and debate about the spiritual challenge of health care and suggests ways forward in implementing spiritual care. It is, perhaps above all, a plea that, in addition to conventional medicine, we need a medicine of a more profound sort that transcends a purely empirical science. Oliver Sacks (1982, p. 253), reflecting upon his experiences, calls these 'a perfectly rational yet practical scientific medicine, and an utterly beautiful and elemental "existential" medicine'. Scientific medicine seeks to rectify the faulty mechanism, the 'It'; 'existential' medicine seeks to inspire the personal, the 'I'. 'These two forms of medicine must be joined, must co-inhere, as body and soul' (Sacks 1982, p. 251).

REFERENCES

Bragan K 1996 Self and spirit in the therapeutic relationship. Routledge, London, p 11

Gadamer H-G 1996 The enigma of health. Polity, Cambridge

Hart D (Written in consultation with Dr Alan Moore) 1997 I swear by the music. Reprinted in The Observer, 6/6/97

Helman C G 1990 Culture, health and illness, 2nd edn. Heinemann, Oxford, p 91

Lyon D 1996 Religion and the postmodern: old problems, new prospects. In: Flanagan K, Jupp P C (eds) Postmodernity, sociology and religion. Macmillan, Basingstoke, ch 1, p 21

Sacks O 1982 Awakenings. Picador, London

Spiritual care, health care: what's the difference?

Julia Neuberger

INTRODUCTION

Spiritual care in the health setting has tended, in the past, to be the speciality of those working in terminal or palliative care. Whilst there has been active chaplaincy in the acute sector (and far too little in the community sector), much of it has been to do with supporting those who are dying or given a terminal sentence within the acute sector, or to do with the support of staff, an enormous part of the chaplaincy role in the modern health service.

But in fact spiritual care goes much wider than chaplaincy. It is not only chaplains who provide it. It is not even primarily chaplains who provide it. It can, and often is, provided by every member of the health care team, if they have the sensitivity and the skills, as well as by other staff members, particularly the cleaning and portering staff, who often, by their very common sense and willingness to talk where health care staff fear to tread, provide some of the best spiritual care in our health care settings in the country.

The conference at which I spoke (Body & Soul, 1996), and on which this chapter is loosely based, is a source of considerable personal pleasure to me. The fact that it was a sell-out, with a waiting list building up within days of the first advertisement, suggests that there are thousands and thousands of people working within the health care setting (and social care, I would argue) who have a need and a desire to talk about the issues of spiritual care, but all too often lack permission to do so. They also often lack a language in which to do it if they are not part of a recognized religious grouping with its own theological language. And that situation, of people having a strong spiritual sense but no conventional religious belief, is something that is increasingly common in our society.

The conference allowed us a chance to begin to develop an agenda which we may wish to take to the NHS as a whole. This is not about the language of contracts, of markets, of outcomes or whatever. This is not the stuff of political debate, largely speaking, nor of party politics. Many managers, hard pressed to provide more and more data with less and less staff (and managers have taken an unfair battering from everyone in recent years and probably need some of the spiritual care themselves) will not see why asking questions about spiritual care fits the agenda of the NHS. Obviously, we cannot be seen to argue for the provision of spiritual care simply because it is 'a good thing', to borrow a label from the authors of *1066 and All That*. Instead, we have to give very good reasons why spiritual care is important. But the doors are beginning to open and people who are clinicians and specialists are beginning to recognize that we, with our view that spiritual care is an important component of health care, may have something to offer.

THE ENVIRONMENT OF THE DEBATE

For the bulk of this century, the view of the medical profession has been that science must take primacy over all else. Thus, we can only do what is scientifically validated or open to validation. This leads to a research-crazy atmosphere, where everyone who is attempting to become a health care professional has to sign up to the view that everything must be proven scientifically (as an article of faith), and therefore everyone in training is now asked to do a piece of research.

The other significant principle readily adopted by all health care professionals, quite rightly, is that we must have evidence-based health care. In other words, it is not enough to practise as we always have, just because that is the way we have always done it. Now, we need strict outcomes measures, strict audit, and to be clear that what we do is effective, and that we do not do things which are damaging to our patients.

Noble aims. It is a very laudable ambition to want only to carry out interventions which are effective. Indeed, the many complex outcomes studies now being engaged in around the country and disseminated by the UK Clearing House on Health Outcomes and the Effectiveness Bulletins, are important. But there are still questions. Only some 20%, if that, of what we do in health care, has actually been shown to be effective. That means some 80% has not been proven effective. It does not mean it is ineffective, but it does mean that nobody has completed an effectiveness study as yet. However, we still carry out those unvalidated procedures, partly, in fairness, because we feel we must do something, we must show patients we have at least tried.

Historically, that has led to such things as fashions in, say, the removal of children's tonsils, or in grommets. It has led to many dilation and curettage operations, arguably utterly unnecessary. And it has probably led to too many hysterectomies. Yet that is the way we do things in Britain, and each country seems more culturally than scientifically driven in much of its health care, despite the emphasis on research.

And we have chaplains. They are there to provide the spiritual care. Historically, they have played a significant role in providing rituals for patients, particularly near death. And nurses have been, historically, those who provided the 'care' for patients, listening to them, getting to know them, soothing fevered brows, being there for them — many of the things we would now class as a form of spiritual care.

THE MODERN SCENARIO

But as things have changed, many nurses find themselves unable to give that kind of attention to patients. They are too busy with tasks. Much of health care is task-driven these days. Health economists and accountants have destroyed what was once often a very caring environment (though it was also often anything but!). If every action is measured, if the pressure is always to reduce costs, to downgrade nurses and have more health care assistants, it is difficult to allow nurses to carry on with the sort of contact with patients that gives them real care, holistic care — spiritual care. There simply is not the time.

Add to that the huge amount of research being done by students and practitioners, and the result, unsurprisingly for the outsider, is that a great deal of not very good research is done by health professionals in training, on the basis that they must learn research methodology. The effect is not at that stage to improve the sum of human knowledge, but rather to invade the privacy of patients to a quite alarming extent, by asking them all sorts of relatively intrusive questions. For asking questions can be as damaging as giving drugs or other invasive treatments, yet most health care professionals fail to see it that way. To be asked intimate details about one's sex life, or bladder control, in a crowded outpatients' department is not, for most of us, an edifying experience. Nor, though most of us wish to help young professionals in training, and realize they have to learn somewhere, and on somebody, do we see why we should be subjected to questioning for research, the standard of which is itself questionable.

Yet this is the scientific method. By taking a statistically significant sample of people, one can ask them certain things and find out, using proper research methodology, something about how they think, or move, or feel. The flaw in this, excellent though it is pedagogically in the teaching of research skills, is that much of it involves asking questions of individuals, without being really interested in the answer as given by a particular individual. In other words, instead of serious concern about the welfare of an individual, and genuine concern about how a fellow human being is feeling, even how they are suffering, the interest lies in getting data for research, in order to get further useful information to help us treat further generations of human patients better.

Yet one is left with the awful feeling that the person in front of one, of whom one has been asking these intimate questions, has just ceased to matter, is not another feeling, sentient human being like the researcher him or herself. A bit of tender loving care, a sign of genuine interest in the wellbeing or otherwise of a particular patient, would be infinitely preferable to the invasion of their space for research reasons. Here, instead of providing health care which is also a form of spiritual care, caring for the whole person as a real human being like oneself, the scientific method much adulated within the health care setting can militate against genuine human contact and continued concern for an individual's wellbeing.

So, if we agree that the only way we can provide effective health care is by specializing, so that people achieve excellence in one particular area, we need to do something to ensure that they acquire excellence in another field of health care, human sympathy, and the care for the whole person that comes with it — something akin to, if not in fact, spiritual care.

And so we get our gastroenterologists, cardiologists, neurologists and so on. Much of what they do is very effective and highly skilled. Most of us want that degree of skill. But that method of qualification and specialization misses out one other thing: anybody who has ever tried to get treated when they have got two things wrong with them at the same time, quite apart from any spiritual needs they may have, knows that if you are there under a gastroenterologist, it is very hard to get your foot dealt with at the same time.

THE WHOLE PERSON

Now, if you take that further, and think that if you need the gastroenterologists, it is probably because you have a severe gastric problem, or if you need the neurologist, it is probably because of your head, then most of us are only too aware that the rest of you does not function all that well either. Your whole being seems to centre on your stomach, or your head, and it stops the rest of you working. Most of us as ordinary individuals find it remarkably hard to disaggregate our head or our knee or our stomach. We do not see ourselves as made up of bits, even if the health care professionals read us that way.

That truth is becoming increasingly recognized within medical and nursing training. And that recognition gives us an opening in this whole debate. We are actually *whole* people and we need to be recognized as whole people. Hence training, and then practice, for health professionals should recognize that wholeness and respond to it, including recognizing our need for spiritual care, when appropriate, and realizing it is not just the premise of another 'specialist', the chaplain. Some of it is ordinary human sympathy and recognition of concerns above and beyond whether one's bowels have been open or whether one has got an oozing wound, and are to do with suffering, pain of a more than physical nature, relationships with family and friends in a state of illness, concerns to which most of us, whatever our discipline, should be able, at the very least, to make a first response.

HOW COULD WE HELP?

One of the changes we have seen come about in the NHS is the system whereby we have named nurses. There is much more recognition than there was ten years ago that individuals in the beds in the ward, albeit there too fleetingly very often to get to know them, unless they are chronically ill and keep reappearing, are people with an identity and a personality and a spirit and a soul, and that they may have needs beyond the fact that they are the gastric case in bed No. 7. So that is our opening: that as whole people, we require a different kind of care.

We do, of course, require the science and the research base. It is important to reiterate the point that no one should think that those of us interested in spiritual care think that the science doesn't matter, because it does! We absolutely should not be prepared to go down the road of 'quackery', of forms of alternative therapy that are not scientifically validated and where people describe themselves as healers without qualification or regulation. There is a side of so-called 'spiritual care' that runs the risk of being just this. The laying on of hands by 'healers' may give some people confidence, but there is little, if any, evidence that it does anything beyond making the individual feel that they are having attention paid to them, and, indeed, being touched.

In fact, there is some suggestion that simply touching people may itself have a healing effect, and our reluctance to touch patients, put a hand on a brow or give a hug or whatever, may lead us into danger of a different kind. If we wish to emphasize spiritual care, we might also wish to include with it the need to recognize that some patients may wish to be touched, within clear rules forbidding intimate touching or abuse of patients, and that recognizing the need for touch is something we could do to improve the quality of *spiritual* care offered to people in our health care settings. For we have licensed touching, by physiotherapists, for example, which is much loved by patients. It makes them feel better, even though the treatment often cannot cure, only alleviate, the condition concerned. But people do not feel better only because their hip has eased, or their knee. They somehow feel better as a whole person, because through touching, and massaging, and comforting, their whole being has been recognized.

But unless we think that there is any evidence of benefit beyond that of simply touching, and paying attention, in a form of care, we should be very wary of it, exactly as we should be wary of those kinds of conventional care which are unproven for efficacy. The two theories go together. We should not do what is not beneficial, and we should do what is helpful: but alongside this we need to recognize that the patient's view of what is helpful and supportive may be different from that of the health economist, or the manager, because often what is helpful and supportive is not easily measurable — just like spiritual care!

But we need to be careful. Evidence of the benefit of acupuncture is now well established. Evidence supporting chiropractic, homeopathy, and osteopathy is mounting, and most of these are now on offer in some way in the NHS. Aromatherapy can be beneficial to people for whom conventional treatments have simply run out, such as those with terminal illness. And we need to think hard about other forms of complementary and alternative therapies, because we need to be as hard on ourselves as people who believe in the value of spiritual care as we are on those who are totally wedded to the scientific approach, without a human face, that has sometimes damaged people as well as helping them. And we need to be clear that when people talk about spiritual healing they mean very different things, some of which are deeply dangerous — and we should have no time for that.

SO WHAT DOES THE FUTURE HOLD?

The scientifically validated or that open to be validated, the effective, the helpful, the compassionate, are all part of what we need to think health care is about, because the scientifically validated or that open to be validated is not all that health care requires. Nurses know this, despite observations and checking drips and pumps, because most of what they offer, most of the most important work that nurses will tell you they do as much as they can, is talking to patients, and, perhaps more importantly, listening to them at moments of great distress, or life change: birth, death, disability, mental breakdown.

This does not only take place in hospital. Indeed, the contact between health professionals and people is more and more in the community. The so-called 'spiritual specialists', the chaplains, are even less available in the community than in the acute hospital setting. Yet here are people who are experiencing all these life-events which have implications about the way people view themselves, their bodies, their health, and their lives.

In mental illness, for instance, now mostly dealt with in the community, people are often searching for meaning, and often cannot even find the words with which to do it, because in this country we have become impoverished in the vocabulary of what we would describe as spiritual care. Spiritual needs are often expressed by those with mental illness, yet how rare it is to find those who work in the field of mental health who are able, or have the time, to respond to that concern, to that need.

Very recently I was talking to one of our patients who had had a major breakdown, and he was describing how, when he started to talk to his family about how he was looking for meaning in his life, they kept on saying to him: 'Stop talking about meaning and go and get a job. Don't be so ridiculous'. Although he pointed out that he was not able to get a job because he was in no fit state to go out, and that meaning in life was very important to him, they ignored him. Yet he felt that, unless he could find meaning, he would not be fit to work anyway.

Some of our staff were trying to help him, as were various parish clergy around the area. But few clergy have real training in working with the mentally ill, though they have a natural sympathy, and few health professionals in mental health have the skills necessary to deal with the spiritual needs of many mentally ill people. Yet here must be a classic case of a need for training, for the clergy, in how to manage people with mental illness in some circumstances, when things sometimes get rough.

Meanwhile, for mental health professionals, who may have some of the skills needed to deal with the tough times with mentally ill people, some training in providing spiritual care — indeed, some training in what spiritual care means — would be very helpful.

For, what we have now cannot be a sensible way to provide care for people who have mental illness. There has been much criticism of 'community care' on the basis that it fails, all too often, to really look after those who are ill. Too many of our mentally ill people are homeless, and feel unsafe. Too many of them fail to take their medication, which is often very unpleasant, and therefore become ill again. Yet there are spiritual needs which many mentally ill people express, and we should be able to devise a way of offering that care, to people within the acute setting and to people within the community.

Reflecting again on the young man whom I met in one of our services in my NHS Trust, he had serious concerns. Yet it was all too apparent that his family thought he was 'crazy', that this was just another feature of his illness, which was driving *them* mad, and that, within families, and within the sort of society we have created, people are quite able to disregard those sorts of questions about meaning, and the meaning of life, until there is some major life-event, like a breakdown, or someone facing death.

Yet, in that situation, an offer of some form of spiritual care, not just by bringing in the chaplain, but by all our staff being aware of where those needs might lie, is terribly important in the way we offer care, and may lead to more effective care in the long term.

But it will require partnerships in the community with other providers of care in social services and the voluntary sector who understand the language of spiritual care as much as they do the language of social care, or hospital care, or community care. It is this language of spiritual care that needs to be in the debate, so that what should be a normal part of anybody's care, anywhere in our health and social care system, can be recognized and discussed.

SPIRITUAL CARE FOR THE TERMINALLY ILL

When it comes to facing death we have a very good record. The hospice and palliative care movement has a very good record of whole-person care, helping people to come to terms with their terminal illness and forthcoming death, and recognizing spiritual issues and needs (see Ch. 12). In most training for palliative care and for those working within hospices, there is considerable emphasis put on spiritual care. Some would argue that there is too much. For a few people, the atmosphere of a hospice is overwhelmingly holy, and somehow unnatural. A friend whose mother died in a hospice recorded how much she hated it, in a private conversation. 'You were somehow, despite all they *said*, not allowed to be angry. It was all just so accepting, so spiritual, so abnormal for most ordinary people.' That is, of course, the converse of recognizing spiritual needs. Not everyone has a clearly expressed spiritual need, and by no means everyone wants these issues to be addressed. There are people who want those questions about the meaning of life, even as they face their deaths, to be left unasked, unconsidered. And there are those who prefer health care to be about physical health only, with a clear boundary between the care of the body and the care of the whole person. We ignore that section of the population at our peril.

But, on the whole, hospices and the hospice movement, the palliative care teams which have grown out of hospices, provide a wonderful service and blend physical and spiritual care together in such a way that one could ask, in terms of this chapter, 'Spiritual care, health care: what's the difference?' But there is a problem with all this; most people don't die in a hospice or with a palliative care team. Even now, most people still die in hospital, and many of them go into the 'old style' caring for the dying, despite all sorts of education and government circulars to change this situation: being put into a side room, and left to get on with it. Drugs are provided. Even in the worst cases, pain control for the terminally ill is far better than it used to be. But only pain control is better. All too often, everything else is ignored. Spiritual needs, emotional needs, the need just for company, the need to ask questions — all these needs are still frequently ignored when someone is dying in a district general hospital.

For hospitals used to be thought of, and sometimes still are, as places for curing people, not for looking after them when they are dying. All the training of young doctors and nurses was and often still is geared towards getting people better, not to alleviating their pain and discomfort when they can no longer improve. Patients who are dying are all too often shoved into a side ward, given a massive dose of morphine every four hours, and left to get on with it. Little was, and sometimes still is, done to alleviate their distress. All too little was and is understood about their pain — physical, spiritual and emotional. Though cruelty was not, and is not, intended, it still takes place every day.

To be packed away and left to die alone, in pain, is a terrible experience for anyone. In a culture where, for most of this century, people have not been talking about death any more, it is cruel. Dying people were often not even told that that was what they were doing. They were given false reassurances in blustery, jolly voices: 'Oh, you'll soon be out of here ...' (in a box ... !); 'We'll get you up and about in a jiffy ...!' (not bloody likely). But the prevailing attitude was not to talk. So the dying person would lie there, high as a kite on morphine for a couple of hours, and in pain, disoriented, without anyone to tell him or her honestly what was happening, with a few people coming in from time to time to talk about the weather — but nothing that mattered.

To some extent, this remains the case, but happily such practice is diminishing. Yet, even now, where a person cannot die in a hospice or at home, staff in hospitals unintentionally treat dying patients in a cavalier way. In many cases, they have not been trained to do otherwise. The ethos of many teaching hospitals is, in any case, to go for acute intervention rather than skilled care of people who in some sense have 'no hope' in the terms of cure-motivated health professionals. Indeed, it is further complicated by the fact that people with very little chance of recovery, or even of remission and survival for any length of time worth talking about, are subjected to heroic interventions, which may be more for the benefit of the carers than of the patients. If carers themselves, health care professionals, have been brought up like the rest of us, then, unless they have been trained specially, they will be unfamiliar with death, even now in hospitals, and regard it as their duty to try to avert it — rather than welcome it, making the patient comfortable in the process.

Yet alongside the development of techniques for keeping people alive, with the great advances in clinical medicine, came the development of the modern hospice movement. Founded in Britain by Dame Cicely Saunders, O.M., it has had a profound effect worldwide. For the modern hospice movement preaches pain control at the very beginning, and then caring for the whole person, not just the physical symptoms. It preaches care, and love, and faith. It is truly about spiritual care, but in the process it offers the best of health care, promoting the wellbeing of those for whom acute interventions are pointless, or not desired, those who are terminally ill, but still alive.

For those without faith, its philosophy can be hard to take. For those who prefer to think of themselves as autonomous individuals with the right to take their own lives, or ask others to take it for them, the hospice is curiously fatalistic. They prefer more decisive action, less prayer and faith. But for many people who do not share the intensity of Christian faith which Dame Cicely Saunders has, as do many of those working in the hospice movement, there is nevertheless much to be gained out of the skilled control of pain developed by the hospice movement, with the proper use of analgesic drugs, indeed often in smaller quantities than conventional hospitals. The philosophy is one of relief of pain, allowing the person to go smoothly and painlessly into death, and treating the whole person: mind, body, spirit, soul. Even those who have no faith are given spiritual care, if they want it.

The hospice movement has had a powerful impact. But it is by no means enough. Fewer than 5% of people die in hospices. More now die at home, around 25%, and many of them with home care teams helping and supporting them and their carers. But there still needs to be more done to challenge the hi-tech view of death, the way that interventions are carried out, and the way caring for dying people in a regular hospital is often so disappointing. The task facing all health care professionals when dealing with dying people is to try to come to terms with the fact that many people do not want all the heroic efforts in the world to be done for them. They do, however, want to be made comfortable, and to be listened to, and cared for as a whole person — and that, with the skills now available and the huge knowledge base about pain control which has been developed as a result of the hospice movement, is entirely possible. And they want dignity to the last.

As death becomes a subject which is easier to talk about and write about, it should be easier to be honest and give people their dignity. It should be easier to have discussions about what people really want at the end of life, how they want to die, whom they want around them, how the health care professionals can provide the best support of all kinds, and, indeed, how the modern skills of life-preservation and of pain control can be used to greatest and most welcome effect.

When that comes about, we will have rehumanized and, indeed, demedicalized, death. Death will happen in our homes, with us there holding the hands of our dying family members. It will happen in the presence of children. It will be considered as normal as it once was, not something one has to leave home to do. There will be expert professional help available, with Macmillan and other hospice home care nurses, with people who can give families a break, who know how to alleviate pain and discomfort, who can provide support of all kinds, including emotional and spiritual care, but they will come to the home. Or be available within a hospice setting, or even a hospital, for those who cannot die at home, or those who do not want to, depending on the ability of their families to care for them. It will be a great tribute to the thinking behind the hospice movement, and the courage of many health care professionals, if this comes about. But, if we are to die well, we must be given the choice of dying at home, with support from professionals, without pain, and with our families around us. We must also be allowed to die in our way, whatever that might be.

For many health care professionals, that is a concept difficult to grasp. But different cultures and religions have very different attitudes to how they wish to die, and to how they wish grief to be expressed, and those differences are important, and can make a huge difference to the wellbeing and comfort of individual patients. That knowledge, the ability to provide individuals with the death they want, within certain parameters, should enable us to have a good death, where and how we want it. It should also enable us to use the experience to show others there is nothing to fear. What we are doing is shedding this life, in a peaceful manner. No mysteries, no horror, no agony. Instead, a peaceful end, as we want it, in as conscious a partnership as possible with those who have been one's life's companions and friends, supported by professional care provided by people with great skill in pain relief and emotional and spiritual support. Then one could truly ask: 'Spiritual care, health care: what's the difference?'.

OTHER AREAS OF SPIRITUAL CARE

Another example where spiritual care and health care intermingle is that of facing new life. Those of us who have gone through the process of pregnancy and childbirth know that, with hormonal changes taking place, there is often a change, even if fairly temporary, of personality. There is wonderment at the miracle of new life, and admiration, and thanksgiving, for perfect tiny hands and feet, for a newborn baby of extraordinary delicacy and beauty. Yet the post-birth 'blues' are more than about something purely physical, although that is often how new mothers are treated. There are questions that we ask about the meaning of our lives at the point of childbirth, or about what kind of world we are bringing our children into. Yet these questions, genuine spiritual concerns for many new mothers, are very poorly taken up in a health care setting. There is clearly a role here for midwives, nurses, and others — and a real task for those psychiatrists and others who deal with the not-uncommon serious postnatal depression.

But when it comes to facing handicapped new life, and many have to do that, although there may be moral discussion as to whether that child should be allowed to live, or whether the mother should have an abortion, very little is done to discuss what the meaning of that life might be, what the value to society as a whole, to the family concerned, and to the child, of that life might be. Yet for many new parents facing that child, and worrying about its future and their own wellbeing, it is those concerns, about meaning and hope, which are foremost in their minds. But our largely utilitarian health care system does not encourage such questioning, even though many parents in that situation would welcome an expression of that kind of concern from professionals involved, and from other parents.

This is not only the province of the religious and religion. I can say that as somebody who is a rabbi, who has even been an acting Protestant chaplain in an American hospital. It is not only the province of chaplaincy. Indeed when you watch what goes on in hospitals and wards, the people to whom patients are actually talking about the things that concern them are mostly the cleaning staff and the nursing staff.

The cleaning staff play a major role in providing spiritual care, and they are not recognized for doing it. One of the reasons it happens that way is that they are there, around the beds and the wards, with their mops, and familiar to patients, unthreatening, in a way that the chaplaincy team cannot be. It is very difficult for chaplains, who are in short supply, to be able to be around sufficiently for the ordinary conversations that then lead on to the important ones. It is much more likely to be a more official visit. Even if it is not intended, that is how it is likely to be perceived. We have to recognize the role that a whole team of caring staff can play in providing spiritual care. And chaplains can often be the trainers and leaders, helping others to recognize real spiritual need, and helping caring staff to ask questions and listen to answers with a trained ear, hearing people's most intimate concerns.

That is all the more important as we realize more and more that for many of our patients in hospitals and in the community, there is no particular religion. When we were setting up home care for the North London Hospice, the first interfaith hospice in the UK, we were terribly keen on providing a multifaith chaplaincy service. We were rather crestfallen when the only person people wanted to see was the Unitarian minister, who was happy to take all comers. For people at home who are religious usually have their own ministers, whilst the others did not want someone with a label attached to them.

Yet they did want something, as most of us tend to on some occasions, whatever the state of our religious faith, or lack of it. In our multicultural society, a new kind of spiritual endeavour has been introduced by Buddhists and Hindus and others, where meditation and contemplation play a particular role. When we talk about spiritual care, there may be things we can learn from people who have a different perspective from the Judaeo-Christian model of chaplaincy, which we could draw into our health care model in just the same way as we can draw in the kinds of health care, such as acupuncture, that come from traditions very different from our own.

CONCLUSION

This agenda for action in spiritual care is an enormous one, which the conference only began to address. Yet it is exciting that such interest has been shown in these issues, and refreshing to see health professionals, managers, cleaners, and porters, alongside patients and carers, able to take on an area of concern together, in a truly interdisciplinary way. If we can integrate spiritual care into all health care, as an option, and get chaplains to be leaders and trainers and supporters rather than the ones thought of as the 'spiritual care specialists', then the environment in which we provide health care will be a healthier one, emotionally, spiritually, and perhaps physically as well.

REFERENCE

Body & Soul Conference 1996 Derbyshire Royal Infirmary NHS Trust, Derby, UK

The meaning of spirituality in illness

Peter Speck

INTRODUCTION

The advent of the Patient's Charter and the issuing of guidelines on spiritual needs by the UK Department of Health (1992) serve to recognize the importance of belief and culture in the lives of many people and especially when they become ill, even if that belief system is non-religious. Most studies of non-medical influences on outcome of acute illness have focused on social and psychological factors (Greer, Moorey & Watson 1989). There has been little research into the possible influence of religious, spiritual or philosophical beliefs on illness except in relation to terminal care, and hospice in particular (Hay 1989, Kirschling & Pittman 1989, Pressman et al 1990, Sherrill, Kaplan & Larson 1989). One reason is the difficulty in measuring the strength and influence of a belief system. Studies have either foundered on problems of definition regarding the concepts being measured, or have simply estimated the strength of spiritual belief in terms of religious activity such as church attendance. While the latter might be one measure of religious practice it is not necessarily an indication of strength of spiritual conviction or spiritual need, as the situation in Box 3.1 illustrates.

THE DEFINITIONS OF 'SPIRITUAL' 'RELIGIOUS' AND 'PHILOSOPHICAL'

The *Oxford English Dictionary* defines *spiritual* as 'The breath of life which gives life to the physical organism' and is, therefore, understood to be a vital principle of humankind. We may not be conscious of its presence or perceive it as an area of need at all times. The outward expression of this vital force or principle will be shaped and influenced by life experience, culture and other personal factors — thus spirituality will be unique for each individual. It may be understood as more than simply a search for meaning, but a search for *existential* meaning within the

---

Box 3.1   Case study

Mavis was a 36 year-old single lady who had discovered that she had breast cancer. She had had several courses of treatment and had now been readmitted to hospital with severe pain in her back, which looked as if it might be related to her cancer. She was frightened and withdrawn. At the time of admission she had told the nursing staff that she was not religious and asked them to put her down as 'agnostic'. During the course of a routine visit to the ward, the hospital chaplain met Mavis. He introduced himself to her and she told him that she 'wanted nothing religious. However, if you can listen, I need to talk to someone non-medical'. Having disavowed her need of anything religious she then invited the chaplain to sit down and began to share some of her worries and anxieties. There were anxieties about her future and whether the pain signified the spread of the disease and what this meant for her life. Why had she become ill in the first place and why at this point in her life when things were going so well? She said that she tried to be realistic about events in her life and so how could she make the best of this situation? If she was going to die what would it be like and what help was available to her? These and many other questions indicated a deep searching for meaning and understanding of her illness, together with a desire for hope for her future and the recognition that she needed to marshall the necessary coping skills in order — as she put it — to 'do it well'. In spite of her definite wish for 'nothing religious', she seemed to be undertaking a very clear 'spiritual' search within the experience.

---

particular experience or life event, with reference to a power other than the self. We may not, however, wish to use the term 'God' to describe the power but may talk about natural or cosmic forces, a sense of the other, a power in the universe, etc.

Spiritual: A search for existential meaning within a life experience, with reference to a power other than the self, which may not necessarily be called 'God'.

A *religion* may be understood as a system of faith and worship which expresses an underlying spirituality. This faith is frequently interpreted in terms of particular rules, regulations, customs and practices as well as the belief content of the named religion. There is a clear acknowledgement of a power other than self, usually described as 'God'. There is a long history of inter-relatedness between religion, healing and medicine.

When talking about religion one would not usually separate religion from spirituality, but neither should one use these terms interchangeably nor assume that people who deny any religious affiliation therefore have no spiritual needs.

Religious: A particular system of faith and worship expressive of an underlying spirituality and interpretive of the named religion's understanding of 'God'.

For some people the search for existential meaning will take a *philosophical* pathway and exclude any reference to a power other than themselves (e.g. existentialism/humanism/atheism). Life events will be interpreted by the individual as a product of the individual's own personality and influence. Atheism, which is the denial of the existence of God, should be distinguished from agnosticism which allows for a degree of uncertainty as to whether or not God exists.

Philosophical: Where the search for existential meaning excludes any reference to a power other than the person themself. Life events and the destiny of the individual being seen as manifestations of the individual's own personality as expressed individually and corporately.

A wider understanding of the word spiritual, as relating to the search for existential meaning within any given life experience, allows us to consider spiritual needs and issues in the absence of any clear practice of a religion or faith, but this does not mean that they are to be seen as totally separated from each other (Speck 1988). In Figure 3.1 we have a Venn diagram to illustrate a possible interrelationship between these three belief systems. Thus, all those belonging to the subset 'religious' would belong also to the set 'spiritual'. But those who are 'spiritual' will not necessarily express that in a religious way, and so they need not belong to the 'religious' subset. Similarly, some of those within the philosophical set will also be 'spiritual' and others not. This becomes important when trying to assess 'spiritual' need, since health care staff may incorrectly deduce that those who decline anything religious have no spiritual needs. Frequently, however,

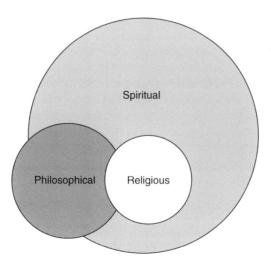

Figure 3.1   Differentiation of 'religious', 'spiritual' and 'philosophical'. Spiritual care is concerned with more than the religious needs of people.

the questions that have been asked only relate to religious practice and need, and so little attempt has been made to explore the spiritual dimension.

In essence we are talking about ways in which people in times of crisis or other formative moments in their life may be aware of a desire to understand or (existentially) make sense of what they are experiencing.

The crisis of illness might introduce the prospect of imminent or untimely death, which certainly triggers off a lot of existential questions for people. In particular, loss and death indicate to people the degree to which they can or cannot exercise control over their lives, their own bodies, the effects of lifestyle, illness and the actions of others. From time to time in our lives we have salutary reminders of this uncertainty which raise questions in the mind which are frequently of an ultimate or existential nature.

The answers to these questions may draw on a belief in a power other than self or not, and there is much variety in the understanding of the nature of that power for those who do hold such a belief system. The power may be attributed to God, or it may be expressed through nature and natural forces. More usually it is expected and understood in the context of a relationship.

The dictionary also defines *spiritual* as a 'vital life principle which integrates other aspects of the person and is an essential ingredient in inter-personal relationships and bonding'. Events which threaten to separate or damage that bond have the potential to threaten our spiritual health and wellbeing. Illness and admission to hospital can have this potential effect since hospitalization may lead to an experience of loss of freedom, independence, bodily function or body part with the consequent impact that such loss has on body image and self-worth (Speck 1978). At times when that bonding is threatened we may feel the event at a very deep level, as if our very existence was under threat. Clearly this is especially so in the event of life-threatening illness. While it is important to respond clinically to the illness, the person will not achieve full health unless he or she is cared for as a whole person and the true impact of the illness explored in both personal terms and in relation to the individual's connectedness with others.

OUR OWN PREPARATION FOR SPIRITUAL CARE

We must endeavour to give sufficient attention to the *whole* person, their coping strategies and sources of meaning and

---

Box 3.2   Case study for discussion of pastoral responses

A 33 year-old married woman (with two children aged 3 and 5) has recently been diagnosed as having leukaemia. She is currently receiving chemotherapy and there is no suitable match for a bone marrow transplant. Her prospects of remission are approximately 50% over three years and she is frightened. She has always had a fear of death ever since she saw a horror movie about a woman buried alive in a coffin. You don't know her but a doctor (member of the Christian Medical Fellowship and your congregation) who works on the haematology team thinks that *you* can help her. He says that she was very weepy when he spoke with her and she told him that she felt 'very let down by God'. She used to be a Sunday School teacher and regular worshipper but it has lost all meaning in recent years. She is, therefore, very critical of God and ambivalent about clergy, but the doctor expects that 'you can deal with that'.

The woman has come home for weekend leave and so is now back in your pastoral area for a brief time.

How would you proceed, and what would you say to her if you visited and, perhaps, to the doctor?

---

strength, if that person is ever to achieve wholeness of body, mind and spirit. This can be difficult to achieve if we have not at times reflected on these issues for ourselves. To share another's journey it can help if one has undertaken some journeying oneself and therefore has some experience of the sort of issues that can arise. Carers can find it difficult to follow the patient's agenda if they find themselves becoming uncomfortable because the patient is raising issues about which they do not feel sufficiently clear. Thus if a patient begins to ask the carer how they make sense of some of the suffering or deaths they witness, they might inadvertently be challenging the carer to share their own uncertainty and discomfort. Sometimes carers find it difficult to say 'I do not know' or 'I do not understand why' since it seems to challenge their self image of being in control and at peace with themselves.

If insufficient attention is given to these wider aspects of the impact of illness then, however fit the person subsequently becomes, they will have achieved a measure of wellness rather than health and wholeness. I believe that we can only achieve this within the context of a personal caring relationship. Such a relationship should create sufficient trust to allow the possibility of journeying together through the experience and to allow the opportunity of exploring together, in order to discover any existential meaning and purpose in the event. This exploration will range over a consideration of the person's life in terms of *Past*, *Present* and *Future* and may identify areas requiring more focused care in relation to guilt, shame, anger, unfairness, vulnerability, hope and confidence in the future (Speck 1997).

Box 3.3 Assessing spiritual needs

This is best done within a caring relationship where it feels safe enough to explore together the experience of the illness in the context of the person's life journey or story. This calls for good observational and communication skills (Stoter 1995) since the exploration should lead to a mutual understanding and the identification of possible coping strategies or options for action. By being attentive to issues relating to Past, Present and Future the carer will begin to identify issues such as:

- *Past*: regrets, guilt, hurt, resentments in need of healing as well as successful events and happy memories to be celebrated.
- *Present*: anger about present situation, frustration and vulnerability. There may also be expressions of helplessness, meaninglessness and loss of control. The carer may also identify current healthy coping strategies and spiritual strength.
- *Future*: issues around hope — realistic and unrealistic — regarding cure or length of life and expectations. Fears of dying and death and 'life after death' may also indicate the need for spiritual support.

In talking about spiritual care in this way the question may arise 'Is this simply "airy-fairy nonsense"; nice for those who believe and find it comforting but not measurable or quantifiable?'. This is not a new question and attempts have been made over the years to research this area and demonstrate the importance of this aspect of care.

ATTEMPTS TO MEASURE THE IMPORTANCE OF SPIRITUALITY

Jarvis & Northcott (1987) surveyed approximately 250 published studies in medicine and epidemiology which included reference to the effects of a religious measure on indicators of a wide variety of causes of mobidity and mortality. Statistically significant associations have been found linking religion and health variables with cardiovascular disease, hypertension, stroke, cancer (especially uterine) colitis, general health status, etc. Regardless of the religious measure used or health outcomes under study, the results are fairly consistent in showing:

1. Comparisons between two or more groups on the basis of religious affiliation show that there is greater health and less mobidity/mortality among adherents of behaviourally strict religious groups (Seventh Day Adventists and Mormons) compared with other religious groups or non-adherents.
2. In studies where religious attendance, subjective religiosity and attitudes were measured, the greater the intensity of religiousness the better was the health and the lower the prevalence of the illness being investigated. This is especially

pronounced for hypertension (Levin & Vanderpool 1987) and in colorectal cancer (Kune, Kune & Watson 1993).

In most of these studies what was being measured was the behaviour of the individual in terms of overt practice of a particular belief system.

The area of study was expanded by Reed (1986) who included the idea of 'well-being'. Terminally ill and healthy adults were compared in terms of 'religiousness and sense of well-being'. Reed defined 'religiousness' as 'the perception of one's beliefs and behaviours that express a sense of relatedness to spiritual dimensions or to something greater than the self'. Wellbeing was defined as 'a sense of satisfaction with one's current life'. In this study, 57 adults in each group were matched for age, gender, education and religious affiliation. The 114 participants completed two questionnaires:

1. The Religious Perspective Scale which was adapted from King & Hunt (1975) and which measures the extent to which people hold certain religious beliefs and engage in religious practices;
2. The Index of Well-Being constructed by Campbell, Converse & Rodgers (1976), which measures satisfaction with life as it is currently experienced.

Women, particularly in the terminally ill group, showed greater religiousness than men. Reed found that both terminally ill and healthy adults indicated moderately high levels of wellbeing and that there was no significant relationship between religiousness and wellbeing in the terminally ill group. Wellbeing was related less to the medical condition than to the ability to engage in activities which give life meaning. In later work, Reed (1987) studied spirituality and wellbeing in terminally ill, hospitalized adults, again matching for age, gender, education and religion. In this later study the confusion between religiousness, spirituality and wellbeing was addressed to *some* extent in that spirituality was defined in terms of transcendence and as 'a broader concept than religion or religiosity'. The results showed a low, but significant, positive correlation between spirituality and wellbeing for the terminally ill, hospitalized adult group. A 'Spiritual Well-being Scale' was devized by Paloutzian and Ellison (1982) to distinguish between the religious and existential dimensions of spirituality. This 20-item measure yields three scores: spiritual, existential and religious wellbeing. The scale was later used to demonstrate that cancer patients with high levels of spiritual wellbeing had lower levels of anxiety (Kaczorowski 1989). However, Kirschling and Pittman (1989) found insufficient evidence to support its validity and reliability.

The possible effect of religion on morbidity and mortality was investigated by Jarvis & Northcott (1987) in relation to various religious groupings: Protestant, Catholic, Seventh-Day Adventist, Latter-Day Saints, Jehovah's Witness, Parsis, Jewish and Muslim followers and clergy. The aim was to go beyond the usual study of the effect of health practices or health-related behaviour, to include social support, religious participation and health-related attitudes. However, their measure of religion depended largely on rates of religious observance. This illustrates the point made in an important review article by Levin and Vanderpool (1987) in which they critically examine the use of 'religious attendance' as a measure of religiosity in epidemiological studies. In their paper they show how the lack of good quality work in this area of study is largely related to a lack of understanding of the language, research methods, and concepts being used by epidemiologists, medical sociologists, theologians and various pastoral workers. There needs to be greater interdisciplinary cooperation in undertaking such studies, in order to address the linguistic difficulties and different conceptual bases, so that a more productive alliance can result (Lukoff & Turner 1992).

Koenig et al (1992) have reported that religious coping was common in hospitalized elderly men experiencing clinical depression. This report was one part of a larger study of depression in hospitalized men; the measure of religious coping was restricted to three questions, two of which measured helpfulness of religious belief and how much the patient used religion to cope.

THE IMPORTANCE OF A BELIEF SYSTEM

For several years Professor Michael King (an academic psychiatrist) and I (as a hospital chaplain) have been collaborating in empirical research to answer the following questions.

- Is it possible for people to describe their belief system, if any?
- Is this belief system in any way predictive of outcome?

Our results have shown that people could describe a belief system (175 out of 300) as religious and spiritual, of whom 172 described a religious faith (King, Speck & Thomas 1994). We also found that patients with a more life-threatening illness were no more likely to express a spiritual or religious view.

Our principal finding was that *strength of belief* (religious and/or spiritual) was more predictive of outcome than scores on the General Health Questionnaire (GHQ) and that those patients who expressed strong beliefs were less likely to do well clinically! This surprising result left us with the puzzling question — Why?

Some possible answers are:

- Impact of diagnostic label varies from patient to patient, but we found no relationship between diagnosis and strength of belief.
- Perhaps strong belief results in reduced fear of death, and therefore people strive less vigorously to live.
- Patients with poor prognosis may focus more on spiritual matters. However, we found the contrary: that strength of belief in those with spiritual/religious outlook had increased significantly at follow-up in those who did well, with little change for others. (This could be due to a cognitive shift during the illness experience.)

We concluded from this preliminary work that empirical study is possible but that care was needed over terminology and the instrument used to measure strength of belief.

DEVELOPMENT AND STANDARDIZATION OF A BELIEF QUESTIONNAIRE

We have since gone on to refine our questionnaire and subject it to test and re-test in order to establish its validity, and it has recently been published (King, Speck & Thomas 1995). It was tested with staff of a large teaching hospital, attenders at an inner-city general practice, and people with a clearly defined, devout, religious belief — in order to establish norms, validity and reliability for each question. It was interesting to note that 71% of hospital staff and 75% of general practitioner (GP) attenders reported a spiritual belief of some kind.

We have since continued our studies and currently have submitted a paper reporting on our main study: 'Spiritual belief and outcome from illness' (King, Speck & Thomas 1997). It is interesting in this study that, out of 250 patients, we once again found that 79% professed some form of spiritual belief, whether or not they engaged in a religious activity. Strong spiritual beliefs were not related to severity of clinical status at admission. 59%

Box 3.4   Some key questions from the Belief Questionnaire

1. I need to understand why things happen to me.
2. My belief helps me during illness.
3. Illness is a result of lack of spiritual belief.
4. My belief is weaker than it used to be.
5. Recently my beliefs have strengthened.
6. Faith in a power outside of oneself is important in healing.
7. Recently I have become less sure of what I believe.
8. Without God I would not have come through my last crisis.

Note: There were five possible responses to each question from 'strongly disagree' through 'strongly agree'. A numerical score of 1 to 5 was allocated to each question, according to the strength of belief. Thus, scores ranged from 8 to 40, with higher scores indicating higher strength of belief with little recent change.

---

were found to be emotionally distressed (on the 12-item GHQ) (Goldberg & Williams 1988), and we also used the Nottingham Health Profile (a standardized quality-of-life scale) and the Social Function Questionnaire (a 9-item measure of social function over the previous 2 weeks).

Once again a strong spiritual belief predicted a poorer outcome at a 9 month follow-up ($p = 0.037$). The only other independent predictor of poor outcome was male gender ($p = 0.029$). Thus strength of belief is more predictive of outcome than clinical state, self-reported impact of illness, or psychological state at admission. The strengths of our studies are:

- the use of a standardized measure of spiritual belief;
- the inclusion of unselected patients;
- a prospective (follow-up) design.

While further work is needed it is clear that patients' efforts to cope in the face of physical illness and hospitalization often incorporate religious beliefs and practices (Whitehead & Stout 1989). This suggests that interventions for improving coping and increased compliance with treatment prescription may be beneficial to the patient (Waldfogel & Wolpe 1993).

CONCLUSION

The results of our empirical studies seem to suggest that patients admitted to hospital who profess strong spiritual beliefs may benefit from an intervention to address this issue in a supportive way since, from our findings, it is *as important* to attend to the spiritual/religious needs as to the psychosocial needs. The reason why strong belief tends to be predictive of poor outcome may be that the content of such a belief system is disturbed or badly shaken by the acute illness, rendering the believer more vulnerable.

A suitable pastoral intervention may enable the patient to restructure the content of his or her belief system and reverse this tendency. In our previous study we found that those with a weak strength of belief at onset of the illness had an increased strength if they experienced a good outcome. There would seem to have been a cognitive shift as a result of the experience. If those tending towards a poor outcome can have access to appropriate spiritual/pastoral support early in the illness experience, it may be possible to reverse the tendency towards joining the poor-outcome group, and further studies are underway to explore this.

Given that strength of belief was more predicitive of outcome than some psychological measures, spiritual care should be a high priority if we are to offer a truly holistic approach in times of illness.

Spiritual care in times of illness is important to patients and should not be neglected. We need to be careful not to assume that, if such beliefs are of little importance to us, they will be of little importance for the patient. If in the course of our exploration of these areas we begin to feel out of our depth, then it is important to seek advice and to liaise with others involved in the care of that person.

The chaplaincy of the hospital or health care trust should be a valuable resource to staff in respect of these issues. Individual chaplains can often offer support and interpretation to staff and patient and, where they cannot supply the need themselves, do have access to others in the local community who can advise as appropriate. Local clergy in the community can also be a valuable resource to health care professionals working within the community, provided a good working relationship can be developed to allow for multiprofessional working.

Many would echo the words of the Prince of Wales, who, when commenting on the architecture of many health care settings at a conference, spoke about not neglecting the soul (or spiritual aspect) of those seeking health and wholeness.

It can't be easy to be healed in a soulless, concrete box with characterless windows, inhospitable corridors and purely functional wards. The spirit needs healing as well as the body.

REFERENCES

Campbell A, Converse P E, Rodgers W L 1976 The quality of American life: perceptions, evaluations and satisfactions. Russell Sage Foundation, New York

Department of Health 1992 Meeting the spiritual needs of patients and staff. HSG (92)2. London

Goldberg D, Williams P A 1988 User's guide to the General Health Questionnaire. Nfer-Nelson, England

Greer S, Moorey S, Watson M 1989 Patients adjustment to cancer: the mental adjustment to cancer (MAC) scale vs clinical ratings. Journal of Psychosomatic Research 33(3): 373–377

Hay M W 1989 Principles in building spiritual assessment tools. American Journal of Psychiatry 147: 758–760

Jarvis G K, Northcott H C 1987 Religion and differences in morbidity and mortality. Social Science and Medicine 25: 813–824

Kaczorowski J M 1989 Spiritual well-being and anxiety in adults diagnosed with cancer. Hospice Journal 5(3): 105–116

King M B, Hunt R A 1975 Measuring the religious variable: national replication. Journal for the Scientific Study of Religion 14: 13–22

King M, Speck P, Thomas A 1994 Spiritual and religious beliefs in acute illness — is this a feasible area for study? Social Science and Medicine 38(4): 631–636

King M, Speck P, Thomas A 1995 The Royal Free Interview for Religious and Spiritual Beliefs: development and standardization. Psychological Medicine 25: 1125–1134

King M, Speck P, Thomas A 1997 Spiritual belief and outcome from illness. Submitted for publication

Kirschling J M, Pittman J F 1989 Measurement of spiritual well-being in a hospice caregiver sample. Hospice Journal 5(2): 1–11

Koenig H G, Blazer D G, Cohen H J et al 1992 Religious coping and depression among elderly, hospitalized, medically ill men. American Journal of Psychiatry 149: 1693–1700

Kune G A, Kune S, Watson L F 1993 Perceived religiousness is protective for colorectal cancer: data from The Melbourne Colorectal Cancer Study. Journal of the Royal Society of Medicine 86: 645–647

Levin J S, Vanderpool H Y 1987 Is frequent religious attendance really conducive to better health? Toward an epidemiology of religion. Social Science and Medicine 24(7): 589–600

Lukoff D, Lu F, Turner R 1992 Toward a more culturally sensitive DSM-IV: Psychoreligious and psychospiritual problems. Journal of Nervous and Mental Disease 180: 673–682

Paloutzian R F, Ellison C W 1982 Spiritual well-being and quality of life. In: Peplau L A, Perlman D (eds) Loneliness: a source-book of current theory, research and therapy. John Wiley, New York

Pressman P, Larson B, Lyons J S, Strain J J 1990 Religious belief, depression and ambulation status in elderly women with broken hips. American Journal of Psychiatry 147: 758–760

Reed P G 1986 Religiousness among terminally ill and healthy adults. Research in Nursing and Health 9: 35–41

Reed P G 1987 Spirituality and well-being in terminally ill hospitalized adults. Research in Nursing and Health 10: 335–344

Sherrill K A, Kaplan B H, Larson D B 1989 Adult burn patients, religious coping and recovery: classic issues in primary care for psychiatric epidemiology. Paper presented at The Section on Epidemiology and Community Psychiatry, World Psychiatric Association, Toronto

Speck P W 1978 Loss and grief in medicine. Baillière-Tindall, London

Speck P W 1988 Being there: pastoral care in time of illness. SPCK, London

Speck P W 1997 Spiritual issues in palliative care. In: Doyle D, Hanks G
    MacDonald M (eds) The Oxford textbook of palliative medicine. Oxford
    University Press, Oxford
Stoter D 1995 Spiritual aspects of health care. Mosby, London
Waldfogel S, Wolpe P R 1993 Using awareness of religious factors to enhance
    interventions in consultation-liaison psychiatry. Hospital and Community
    Psychiatry 44: 473–477
Whitehead P L, Stout R J 1989 Religion as ego support. In: Treatment of
    psychiatric disorders: a task force report of the American Psychiatric
    Association, vol 3. American Psychiatric Association, Washington DC

The re-enchantment of health care: a paradigm of spirituality

Pamela Reed

INTRODUCTION

It has been said that in this postmodern age, music has done away with melody, cinema with narrative, and art with figuration. Similarly, it has also been said that modern advancements in science and technology have matured society to the point where the health sciences have done away with the spiritual. Scientists and clinicians have therefore been confronted with some critical if not uncomfortable questions. Is spirituality a constructed reality, something inscripted on the human body, a melody contrived to serve ulterior purposes? Or might spirituality in fact be relevant to human health and health care? The purpose of this chapter is to answer this question by proposing an emerging paradigm of spirituality in health care as based upon the conceptual and empirical literature of the past decade.

Theories and paradigms are important in making things matter and in testing the reality and usefulness of ideas. Sloan (1992), an historian, pointed out that science has used quantum theory to make real the infinitely small, and has used relativity theory to make real the infinitely large, leaving underdeveloped theories about the terrestrial world in which human beings actually live. So, to better understand the spiritual reality in the everyday world of health care, and perhaps to make it matter more, an important step is to put forth for discussion and critique a conceptualization of spirituality as generated by current scholarship and research into healing, health care and health experiences. What becomes apparent, in doing this, is that the gods are still a hypothesis of interest among scientists and practitioners in health care.

SPIRITUALITY — AN HISTORICAL PERSPECTIVE

The history of healing reveals a pervasive concern with spirituality in the processes of living and health care practices. In premodern time, learned scholars spoke of souls and spirits that constituted the human being, enlivened and mediated human functions, and connected human health and community life to the heavens. The Aristotelian view connected body and soul like a statue to marble. During the Medieval era, body and soul came to be viewed as two distinct entities; material and spiritual were officially separated in explaining birth, death, life and health. The dissection of corpses and other observations of the human body influenced a strongly materialistic view of human beings during the Renaissance in Europe, while the Indians of North America were celebrating the delicate balance between their spiritual and natural worlds.

During the Enlightenment, what Aristotle had once integrated, Descartes divided. Baconian empiricism and Cartesian notions of divisions between spirit, soul, mind and body ushered in Modern thinking in which sciences grew out of distinctions created between body and soul and, more specifically, between mind and soul. However, modern science, as Reed (1997) explains, was not designed to disprove religious or mystical ideas, but rather to help thinkers avoid conflict between religion and science. The new science of psychology at the turn of the century, for example, replaced a science of the soul with a science of the mind.

Throughout history, however, the relationship between body and soul, and the nature of the human spirit, were important focuses of philosophical debate. Soul and spirit were not only concepts of theology, but entered into scientific concerns. During the time when Descartes elevated the importance of mind and relegated the soul to a place within a pea-sized gland in the brain, the Scottish physician, Whytt, put forth ideas about a soul distributed throughout the body, regulating all critical functions. Charles Darwin entertained hypotheses, later refuted based upon his data, about a higher force at work in evolution.

Even as mechanistic science was taking a foothold in the 17th century, there remained a belief in a spiritual as well as material reality. While positivist psychologists were postulating physical structures within the brain that effected human behaviour, soul psychologists explored naturalistic expressions of spiritual phenomena such as prayers and miracles. Concurrent with the materialism of the Enlightenment, Eastern Hinduism and American individualism combined to influence the transcendental views expressed by Emerson that linked soul and nature. And although medicine and nursing suspended the spiritual elements while pursuing their modernist scientific study of the body, these professions acknowledged existence of moral and spiritual elements in their philosophies of care of human beings.

The New Age movement emerged as an outgrowth of the disillusionment with modern science and in an attempt to reunite body and spirit and tap a universal energy for health and transformative change in the individual and society (Melton 1988). The New Age marked a transition between modernism and postmodernism during the early 1970s.

The postmodern era, dating from the late 1960s to the present, was and still is a time of deconstruction of cherished beliefs about the existence of a single truth and a single method to obtain knowledge about that truth. Postmodernists deconstruct long-held ideals to expose inconsistencies and values that oppress others. Postmodernism attempts to replace the modernist idea of person as a body, possessed of an inner soul or mind as its motivating force, with the new idea of person as a blank slate on which society inscribes notions about health, illness, spirituality, and other discourses (Fox 1994). There is no transcendent reality, the gods have fled. As there is really no melody in music or figurative theme in art, neither is there an inner essence of the person, only what disciplines have created or inscribed onto the human body. Any truths that appear to exist have come about not through a historical evolution toward progress, but as a product of time and change, based upon someone redescribing nature in a way that is temporarily useful to the current culture and context. Spirituality is not an inherent human process, it is a discourse, that is, 'written, spoken, or enacted practices organized by others so as to [provide] a coherent perspective' for some purpose (Fox 1994, p. 161).

SPIRITUALITY — A CONCEPT FOR SCIENCE

People invoke the spiritual to fill gaps in knowledge about the mysteries of the everyday world. There is a paradox in this behaviour in that it effectively blocks understandings about spirituality. First, spirituality is frequently defined in terms that imply its non-existence in the terrestrial world, and imply that perhaps it does not matter in health care. Words such as mysterious, intangible force, numinous, immeasurable, supernatural, ethereal, and — worst — ineffable are used to define spirituality. Granted, each of these words expresses something special about the complexity and depth of being human, but when they are offered up as the definitive descriptors of spirituality, they do not foster understanding. Second, and more significant, is that the word, 'spiritual', is used to label phenomena or events that are believed to exist but are unknowable, unseen, or cannot be explained. It follows logically then, that once phenomena can be explained or 'observed' by some means, they are no longer regarded as spiritual.

Defining the spiritual only in terms of the unseen or the unexplained effectively limits scientific and clinical under-standings about spirituality. As science progresses in its observations and explanations of phenomena, we will come to know less and less about what is designated as spiritual. If the spiritual is defined as ineffable, understandings of spirituality will shrink as knowledge of the knowable grows; for if we can know about it, it must not be spiritual. There is a tyranny in all this — posing spirituality as essential to life, the very breath of being, yet regarding it as something that cannot be known, or measured, or taught.

RESEARCH DOMAINS

A review of the research into spirituality suggests that spirituality can be conceptualized in a way that preserves the mystery while facilitating an understanding of spirituality in health care. Research on spirituality in health care has clustered around what seem to be areas of particular need: aging and mental health; terminal or serious illness; chronic illness; and wellness. The findings from research in these areas suggest that spirituality, as measured in a variety of ways, taps into a human pattern across various health experiences.

Aging and mental health

Research results indicate that a number of spiritual dimensions are significant to mental health in later life. Koenig and his colleagues (1988, 1992, 1995) have published several studies during this decade, which focused on depression and religious coping in men undergoing treatment at the Veterans' Administration hospital. Religious coping was defined in terms of the use of religious means, such as prayer, faith, and drawing strength from belief in God, as strategies to cope with illness. His results consistently supported the finding that men who reported increased religious importance over time were less likely to be depressed and were better able to cope with their life situation. He also found that religious coping was the only baseline variable that predicted lower depression scores in a 6-month follow-up study of 200 men.

Other studies (e.g. Pargament et al 1990, Pressman et al 1990) have indicated that intrinsic religious orientation (whereby the motivational source for religiousness is intrinsic rather than extrinsic to the person) and a collaborative style of religious coping are particularly related to positive mental health outcomes. A collaborative style of coping is that whereby both person and God share in the problem-solving, in contrast to either a self-directed style, which focuses on the person as primary source of responsibility, or a deferring style, by which God is the source and action. From a physiologic perspective and as a result of his research into neuroendocrine and chemical functioning, Restak (1989) has suggested that spiritual resources may alter the links between stress and brain and immune function.

Nursing researchers have studied mental health as related to spirituality. Butcher (1996) conceptualized depression in the elderly as 'dispiritedness', defined as a pattern that emerges when patients state they have lost their spirit, feel low in spirits, or have a broken spirit. These individuals feel detached from life's flow, and have a sense of meaninglessness, constricted self-boundaries, and loss of will and energy. Similarly, Morris (1996) studied the problem and treatments of depression as spiritual distress, whereby the focus is on a disruption in harmonious connections between self, community, nature, and a higher power. Reed (1989, 1991b) and Young & Reed (1995) identified self-transcendence to be a significant correlate of mental health, diminished depression, and wellbeing in elders.

Terminal or serious illness

There is an abundance of literature on spirituality in the terminally or seriously ill. This research domain was a readily accepted area of study in the 1970s and early 1980s when spirituality was breaking into the empirical world of science, which offered a limited repertoire of treatments for these patient populations. As one of the first nurses (allowed) to examine spirituality in doctoral research, Reed (1986a, 1986b, 1987, 1991a) conducted a series of studies. The findings provided empirical support for the salience of spiritual perspective and its relationship to wellbeing among various groups of terminally ill adults, ranging from ambulatory adults who had to carry out their activities of daily living with keen awareness of their mortality, to critically ill adults who were in active stages of dying.

Researchers have identified other expressions of spirituality that are significant in terminal or serious illness, particularly among patients who are openly aware of a terminal prognosis. Findings include that: belief in and a relationship with God, and involvement in religiously oriented activities throughout the day are therapeutic for patients under treatment for cancer (Fehring et al 1997, Sodestrom & Martinson 1987); and that religiously-oriented expressions of transcendence are more important than are existential or psychological expressions of transcendence in women with breast cancer (Mickley et al 1992) and African-American adults with cancer (Potts 1996). Among men and women with HIV/AIDS, there were clinically important healing effects of looking inward and self-reflection in relation to the meaning of life and belief in a higher power (Coward 1990, 1991, Hall 1997). Spiritual and religious involvement were found to have a positive effect on survival among disabled elderly living in the community (Idler & Kasl 1992) and among elderly who had undergone cardiac surgery (Oxman et al 1995). Also found was the positive influence of prayer on emotional coping and physiological outcomes associated with surgery (Byrd 1988, Saudia et al 1991). A significant positive relationship between spiritual involvement and sense of power was identified in long-term survivors of polio (Smith 1995).

Noticeably absent from this domain of research is the study of patients with Alzheimer's disease. Might this dearth reflect a mentalist ontology of spirituality — the view that spirituality resides solely in a normally functioning mind, disconnected from body? Koenig (1993) reported an inverse relationship between cognitive impairment and religious coping. But might there be other spiritual expressions that are salient among those who are cognitively impaired? Clinicians repeatedly report the effectiveness of touch, song, poetry, faithful presence of the caregiver, facial expressions, and other means of expressing spirituality and transcendence with Alzheimer's patients (e.g. McFadden 1996, Muldoon & King 1991). This is corroborated by the personal account of minister Robert Davis (1989) in writing his book about his journey into Alzheimer's disease. Caregivers of Alzheimer's patients have been studied, with findings supporting the significance of a spiritual life perspective among caregiving spouses (Kaye & Robinson 1994), religious faith in God among black family caregivers (Wykle & Segal 1991), and spiritual reframing of the initial hopelessness of the situation (Wright et al 1985).

Chronic illness

Chronic illness is often faced as a journey that has no particular destination nor any clear rest stops. Spiritual issues that arise are related to the challenges that chronic illness presents in terms of societal values about wholeness, independence, normalcy, and vitality. Research indicates that various dimensions of spirituality become salient in different populations of chronically ill patients: existential issues as related to quality of life among long-term cancer survivors (Wyatt & Friedman 1996); religious aspects as related to diminished loneliness among older adults with rheumatoid arthritis (Miller 1985); existential concerns as related to wellbeing among young persons with diabetes mellitus (Landis 1996). In a large epidemiological study of 560 well and chronically ill adults, Michello (1988) found that a relationship with God was a distinctly important factor in the health satisfaction among those who had chronic health problems. Thomas (1989) reported that interventions for hypertension, that helped guide people in contemplating personal philosophy, boosted the healing process in terms of lowering blood pressure and enhancing overall wellbeing.

Research on chronic pain (Conwill 1986) highlighted the spiritual meanings often given to pain by patients, and the importance of integrating these meanings into therapy for chronic pain. Low (1997) identified three spiritual themes predominant in these patients: pain as punishment, as redemptive, and as an opportunity for transcendence.

Wellness

Wellness, as a health experience, has garnered less research attention, although the integrative or holistic models of health care emerging in response to the community-based, managed care models of treatment reflect increasing attention to spirituality. This is not surprising, because spirituality may be used to reduce health problems that generate high health care costs, such as those related to violence, alcoholism and other addictions, other risky behaviours, and prolonged grief (Hilsman 1997, Miller 1997).

Community-based approaches that elicit God as partner in healing and maintaining health are emerging (Bergquist & King 1994, Pargament et al 1990). Similarly, other research with well elders identified the importance of prayer, divine relations, and other religious activities that connect one to God (Kraus & Van Tran 1989, Levin 1996, Levin et al 1995, Musick 1996, Pollner 1989,

Reed 1991b); this is so particularly among older women and older black Americans. More generally, Goddard (1995b) identified the theme of spirituality as an integrative energy in health experiences across various cultures, historically and at the present time.

Emerging themes: spirituality and transcendence

A predominant theme researchers and clinicians have used to distinguish spirituality from other concepts is transcendence, as a connection to or awareness of a transcendent dimension, whether this is God, inner self, or a purpose or other dimension greater than the individual. Elkins (1988) and Ellison (1983), both of whom have developed measures of spirituality, have defined spirituality as a way of being and experiencing life that is based on an awareness of a transcendent dimension. Moberg (1997), a noted sociologist who has studied spiritual wellbeing, presented a definition of spirituality that crosses disciplinary boundaries and emphasizes the transcendent, in citing the National Interfaith Coalition on Aging definition of spiritual wellbeing: 'The affirmation of life in relationship with God, self, community, and environment, that nurtures and celebrates wholeness'.

Similarly, Reed (1992) has defined spirituality in terms of a capacity for self-transcendence that is expressed by expanding personal boundaries intrapersonally, interpersonally, and transpersonally — inward, outward, and upward. Transcendence can be found within or beyond self, depending upon one's religious or philosophical beliefs.

An important perspective within this model of spirituality is that transcendence is a process connected to the body. Research results from the studies reviewed, as well as writings from philosophers and clinicians who work with ill or aging patients, support the idea that embodiment is an important consideration in understanding spirituality (e.g. Olafson 1995, Picard 1997). Human beings are not disembodied spirits or souls. Transcendence is expressed across a diversity of experiences that are embodied yet enable the person to reach beyond their present situation, such as through making meaning, enacting choices, and having mystical or out-of-body experiences.

SOUL AND SPIRIT IN TRANSCENDENCE

From this perspective of spirituality, transcendence is a process of being that is found in both the inner reaches of the soul and the outward reaches of the spirit. Watchman Nee's (1968) ideas, along with others (e.g. Elkins 1995, Helminiak's 1996 interpretation of Lonergan, Hillman 1975), are useful in proposing distinctions between spirit and soul (see Fig. 4.1). Soul, from the Greek translation of soul as psyche, is linked most often to what today is referred to as the person's emotional experiences of awe, meaning, despair, suffering, joy, and beauty. Soul is about depth, whereas spirit is about height (Elkins 1995). Spirit, from the Greek translation 'pneuma' expresses connectedness to a creative power beyond the self, and equips one to commune with God and other spirits (Nee 1968). The soul provides self-consciousness and emphasizes the faculties of volition, intellect, emotion. The spirit facilitates God-consciousness through intuition, mystical experience, or other means of direct knowing.

Research results support the components of soul and spirit in spirituality. Goddard (1995a) examined themes of spirituality shared across several sources: mythological and poetic literature, historical descriptions, aboriginal stories, developmental science, and the clinical and theoretical literature found in the health disciplines. She identified seven categories, three of which relate to spirit transcendence: relationship between humans and God; physical transcendence; and divine immanence. Four categories relate to soul transcendence: relationship to others; connections to nature; personal journey of discovery; and integrative energy within self.

Emblen and Halstead (1993) interviewed patients, nursing staff, and chaplains to identify definitions of spirituality. Six categories were generated across all three groups. Two of these relate to the spirit component of transcendence: religious beliefs and activities, and contact with God. One category, values, related to both spirit and soul, with values such as health, freedom from guilt, hope, faith, and the sacraments. The remaining three categories related to soul: relationships with others; affective experiences (like peace and comfort); and communication abilities.

Ferder's (1982) conceptualization of spirituality as the integration of wholeness and holiness mirrors the two

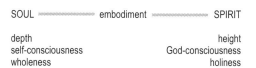

Figure 4.1 Transcendence.

dimensions of transcendence, soul and spirit, respectively. Wholeness emphasizes the roles of mind and body within personal development, self-awareness, and insight into others' needs. Holiness refers to an awareness of a higher power and a relatedness to God. Thus, as soul and spirit both define transcendence, it is the integration of wholeness and holiness that defines spirituality.

A MULTIPARADIGM MODEL OF SPIRITUALITY

The various research studies into spirituality that have occurred over the last decade can be located on a two-dimensional conceptual map or model of spirituality (see Fig. 4.2). The horizontal axis represents an epistemology of spirituality in terms of scientific approaches to knowledge development and ways of knowing, which range from modern to postmodern. The vertical axis represents an ontology of spirituality in terms of ways of being and the spiritual nature of humans. Ways of being

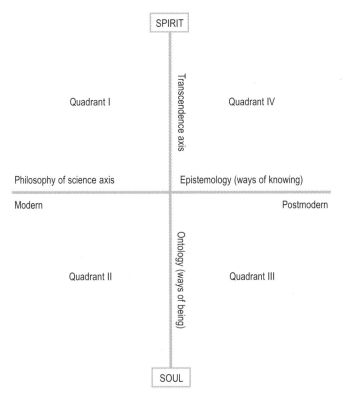

Figure 4.2 A multiparadigm model of spirituality. © Pamela Reed

spiritual are expressed through soul and spirit forms of transcendence.

The model consists of four quadrants, created by the intersection of the two axes. The model presents a diversity of perspectives on spirituality that share the two axes, ways of knowing and ways of being. The various research studies can be organized according to four paradigms, identified by the four quadrants of the spirituality model. Each quadrant represents a paradigm of spirituality, based upon how the research (a) addressed spirit or soul forms of transcendence and (b) reflected a modern or postmodern philosophy of science. Each paradigm's relevance to health care practice is based in part on the extent and nature of the research supporting it.

The four paradigms also represent domains of praxis, that is, a perspective for practising health care in a way that enacts one's values, theories, skills, and research-based knowledge about spirituality. Through praxis, links are made between the values of philosophy, the ideals of scientific research, and the realities of practice (Reed 1995).

Quadrant I

Quadrant I is bounded by a spirit view of transcendence and a modernist philosophy of science. Within this paradigm, spirituality is understood primarily in terms of a dualist view whereby spirituality, as part of mind, affects the body, through religious behaviours and beliefs that can enhance psychological coping. Also, religiousness may serve as protection against mortality and a variety of illnesses by influencing lifestyle choices in foods eaten or avoided, sexual and social behaviours, and use of drugs. Divine action may be believed to exist, but it is not something to study or to use in explaining the functioning of spirituality in health care. Prayer, organized religious participation, and other religious activities may be prescribed as part of the patient's repertoire of health behaviours, with the assumption that religious activities function as cognitive, psychologic, or sociologic mechanisms to enhance coping with the stress of illness.

Scientific explanations of spirituality do not extend beyond these applications of spirituality within this paradigm. Spiritual phenomena, such as when a dying person experiences a visit from a deceased relative, are pathologized or physicalized and may be attributed to hallucinations, anoxia, or the effects of drugs. Prayer is believed to work because of its psychophysiologic effects on the body in terms of enhanced immunity, relief from guilt, and sense of personal control. Beyond these empirical effects, spirituality is considered to exist, though as a supernatural process, and is immeasurable and not within the purview of science. Research generated within this paradigm has produced some important findings.

An analysis of research over the past decade indicates that there is a diversity of studies occurring within Quadrant I. The following are conceptual areas of spirituality, along with the patient population or health experience targeted in research: religious coping among elderly with mental health problems, elders who underwent hip surgery, and the terminally ill; religious beliefs among women with rheumatoid arthritis; religious participation as related to elder survival, quality of life, and depression; spiritual support in caregivers; faith among those receiving haemodialysis and who are caregivers; prayer as coping among those with drug addictions or who are undergoing surgery; and hope among patients with recurrent cancer.

Implications for praxis that are inferred from the findings of these studies focus on strategies to enhance religious coping by supporting the patients' beliefs in spirit-based forms of transcendence. Health care providers would assist the patient in religious practices, express respect for beliefs and rituals, allow for religious rituals, support the patient's faith and hope, and encourage use of prayer and other coping skills.

Quadrant II

Quadrant II is bounded by soul expressions of transcendence and modern philosophy of science. The characteristics of the work generated within this perspective are similar to those in Quadrant I except that here the focus is on mind–body phenomena, particularly the functions of the mind as it affects the body.

Within this paradigm, the spiritual is addressed by calling it mind, soul, or consciousness, and it is operationalized in terms of mental imagery, neurologic mechanisms, attitudes or emotional feelings. The mind affects the body through soul-like emotions, which can trigger psychoneuroimmunologic responses, psychosomatic effects, placebo effects and flow of hormones and other chemicals that affect health. A stunning example can be found in a recent newspaper headline announcing that 'despair speeds heart trouble in men'. The article explained that middle-aged men who feel hopeless or think of themselves as failures may develop atherosclerosis faster than their more optimistic cohorts. This research finding, reported in the August 1997 issue of the American Heart Association Journal, *Arteriosclerosis, Thrombosis and Vascular Biology*, stated that people who expressed high levels of despair had a 20% greater increase in atherosclerosis over 4 years, a risk equivalent to a one-pack-a-day smoker.

Research findings reported during the last decade that fit within Paradigm II cluster under the conceptual areas of spirituality research focused on self-transcendence and elder depression; existential wellbeing among patients with diabetes and others; hope in newly diagnosed cancer patients; and other soul-related dimensions that influence health and wellbeing. Hopelessness, inner conflicts, loneliness, and other expressions related to soul transcendence (or the lack thereof) may also be included in this research domain.

Health care praxis within this quadrant would focus on developing a therapeutic relationship with the patient through which patients could be helped to express feelings, reframe negative thinking, learn stress reduction strategies, and experience emotional support and a sense of self-worth.

Quadrant III

Quadrant III is bounded by soul expressions of transcendence and a postmodern philosophy of science. This quadrant supports humanistic and holistic perspectives with emphasis on the individual, development of self-consciousness, and transcendence of ego. Soul expressions of spirituality permeate the life of the patient, and are not separate from one's physical body as they are within the Quadrant II paradigm. Phenomena are addressed from the person's perspective. Paranormal and mystical experiences are legitimate areas of study, as they are legitimate experiences of human beings. Congruent with field phenomena, the soul is not thought of as in the brain but in the field, with the human being viewed as an energy field (Rogers, 1980). Within this paradigm, for example, caregivers do not have a relationship with patients, they have a presence; self-transcendence is not just a perspective, it is a lived experience; and terminal cancer is not only a disease with specified psychological sequelae, it is an inner journey.

Areas of spirituality research within this third paradigm conceptualize illness as a spiritual experience, as for example, when depression is conceptualized as dispiritedness, or hypertension is related to integrative energy. Other conceptual areas of research identified include: the lived-experience of self-transcendence among those with terminal cancer; the inner journey of terminal cancer patients; depression as spiritual distress, and caregiver presence with persons who have Alzheimer's disease.

Health care praxis within this paradigm utilizes a variety of approaches that focus on nurturing the soul and self-transformation. Fostering 'spiritual serendipity' (Eyre 1997) is one method of cultivating spiritual energy. This is done by learning to more purposefully attend to feelings, events, nudges, impressions, and flashes of insight that help people get in touch with the spiritual in their everyday lives. Other approaches include conveying a caring presence with patients, facilitating soulful awareness, and assisting patients in contemplative and meditative techniques to facilitate spiritual development.

Health care providers may also participate simply by expressing their support, care, and compassion for the patient through the healing process. It is also considered therapeutic for clinicians to inquire about patients' use of alternative techniques, and refer them to spiritual healing practitioners. Alternative therapies may include spiritual healing, therapeutic touch, acupuncture, positive thinking, channeling, and relaxation with an aim of tapping into a rhythmic, universal energy that activates the person's inner healing potential. Many of these techniques are borrowed from the spiritual traditions and practices. An important difference, however, is that the spiritual ideology is split off from the practice (Melton 1988). Like a minimalist approach to spirituality in health care practice, for example, meditation and yoga are practised outside of Buddhist beliefs, prayer without Christian or Jewish beliefs, and faith healing without the traditional faith. These practices, while they may not nurture the spirit, can nurture the soul.

Mechanisms of healing beyond the local conceptions of space and time also are considered within this perspective. They are not thought of as supraempirical or supernatural, but within the realm of reality explained by the new physics; that is, matter may behave as a particle and be present in one place at a time, or it may behave like a wave or field of energy and have non-local effects. Soul-focused therapies, found through art, music therapy, bibliotherapy, and spiritual life review, can be integrated into the patient's treatment plan to facilitate soulful transcendence during illness.

Because body and soul are connected, it is feasible that, through research and practice, scientists and practitioners will make new discoveries about how paranormal phenomena 'participate in patterning bodily functions' such as blood pressure, heart rate, and the flow of substances such as insulin (Phillips 1996). These discoveries may reduce clinicians' dependence on external treatment modalities by offering a basis for a more informed and deliberate practice based upon integration of body and soul.

Quadrant IV

Quadrant IV is bounded by spirit-based transcendence and a postmodern philosophy of science. In contrast to the humanistic or soul-focused forms of transcendence of Quadrant III, the perspective here is theistic or, in the case of Christianity, theotic — a term Helminiak (1996) uses to refer to the three elements of the Godhead in Christianity. Mystical experiences, whereby one has direct awareness of God, are considered legitimate forms of spirituality relevant to health care even though they cannot be readily described.

Within this paradigm, human beings' spirituality in health care is understood in reference to 'an inherent striving to relate to God, and God to human beings' (Koenig 1994). For example, spiritual distress is that in which the patient feels disconnected from God, and aging may be interpreted as a process of increasing spiritual awareness. As in the third paradigm, paranormal phenomena are considered legitimate experiences, but they will be linked to God or spirit, rather than soul experiences. Spirit visitation and other mystical experiences, for example, may be considered a normal part of dying and bereavement. Human and Divine participate in a spiritual process that is explained either through natural laws, supernatural explanations, or laws of nature not yet discovered.

Conceptual areas of research are those in which spirituality is expressed in relation to spirit or God. Areas of research during the past decade that define this paradigm include: spiritual distress in depression; relationship with God among those who have a chronic illness, Alzheimer's disease or cancer; divine relations in well populations; prayer in elder mental health and those in coronary care; pain as redemptive among those physically disabled; spirit visitation during bereavement; and intrinsic religious orientation as related to cardiac surgery survival, polio survival, cancer outcomes, and wellness.

Health care praxis within this paradigm focuses on nurturing the patient's spirit and spiritual gifts. This may entail designing experiences and environments in which patients can commune with God, celebrate their relationship with God, and continue to grow spiritually. Allowing or creating time for patients to express spiritual needs or for receiving the sacraments with clergy are also important practices within this paradigm. Aldrich (1993) expressed the clinician's focus succinctly in saying that it all comes down to an 'interest in understanding how patients who come to us for healing see their problems in the context of their relationship with God' (p. 83).

THE RE-ENCHANTMENT OF HEALTH CARE

Scientists and health care providers, like artists and philosophers, have perceived the need for a re-enchantment of the professions by integrating notions of the sacred that existed earlier in the history of healing. Elkins (1995) and Reed (1997) in psychology, Aldrich (1996) in medicine, and Rogers (1980) and Newman (1995) in nursing have all called for a new paradigm in which the phenomena of each discipline are studied from a holistic perspective. This perspective embraces spirituality as a lived and embodied experience of transcendence across a diversity of health experiences. Rather than correspond only to abstract ideas about truth, paradigms must relate to the embodied and contextual sources of truth — the personal experiences and wisdom of the local context. The Indian philosopher, Chatterjee (1989) wrote, 'Much talk of the spiritual tries to provide a grammar of ascent, whereas it is in the horizontal dimension that we must walk from day to day' (p. 102). The spiritualities of persons experiencing chronic illness, terminal illness, acute illness, or wellness may differ as well as share significant patterns. This calls for a multiparadigm view of spirituality in health care; it is a perspective that allows for an ongoing hermeneutic whereby persons and their families can reinterpret the spiritual self as illness and health experiences alter their lives (Aldrich 1996). The new model of spirituality in health care that has been presented here is not a singular paradigm. Rather, the review of the literature revealed spirituality to encompass a diversity of discourses about transcendence — from the inner journey of the soul to a reaching beyond to God and other spirits. The empirical research and other literature presented varying ontologic and epistemologic perspectives.

Unlike 'superego' or 'synapse', the concept of spirituality was not invented by any single discipline. Because of this, the concept of spirituality is more responsive to the pluralism of postmodern thought. Postmodernism opens up many possibilities for understanding spirituality — from traditional narratives to those more futuristic. Research results indicated that traditional religious beliefs and behaviours are not anachronistic, and continue to have meaning for significant numbers of patients. New Age spirituality has not supplanted old-time religion. Traditional religious practice can reveal human nature's basic, if hidden, connection to a transcendent order (Murphy 1992, p. 549).

Nevertheless, the new physics, quantum theory, and repeated occurrences of mystical and other extra-ordinary phenomena have implications for understanding spirituality (Levin 1996, Murphy 1997, Rogers, 1980). Griffin (1997), for example, anticipates a new way of knowing in the study of spirituality in which religious experience may be attributed either to soul or to spirit forms of transcendence — that is, for example, attributed to influences of one's imagination, personal desires, beliefs, or to direct encounters with God and spirit.

However, if our models of spirituality do not account for these possibilities, we will not be able to discover them in research or assess them in practice. Researchers, for example, who are careful to avoid 'being limited by specific theologic issues' in spirituality (e.g. Carson & Green 1992) may need to transform their paradigms to accommodate the diverse forms of spirituality currently found among persons receiving health care.

CONCLUSION

The clear boundaries between pastoral care roles and health care roles that existed with distinctions between religion and science in the modern era, become more blurred as spirituality is integrated into health care (Brittain 1986, Post 1997) in the postmodern era. Today, those in health care settings who give attention to spirituality cannot necessarily be distinguished by the clothes they wear. Where once hospital chaplains and clinicians kept their values about health and healing separate, today medicine is embracing religion as a 'twin healer' and nursing is regarded in part as spiritual care. Still, it is not likely that any one role will be usurped by another. With increased research-based knowledge about the importance of spirituality, health care providers will better understand the complexity of spirituality and will see a need for even more involvement of pastoral care in health care, as well for the integration of the spiritual dimension in health care overall.

Horgan (1996) created a stir with his book, *The End of Science*, in which he explained that we are now in the twilight of the scientific age, facing the limits of knowledge. His work reflects the deconstructionist and pessimistic side of postmodernism, and restricts definitions of 'knowledge' to traditional views of 'scientific knowledge'. In contrast, Capra (1996) has put forth a call to reconnect the web of life, and he proposes that this be done by focusing on the mind as the unifying process. I suggest that, instead of mind, spirituality in all its ontologic and epistemologic diversity, be a focus for this unifying process. Spirituality, in a new way, can again rush in to fill the gaps that the 'sacred world of science cannot fill' (Takacs 1996) and re-enchant the science and practice of health care. Twilight is dawn.

REFERENCES

Aldrich D 1993 Patients and their spiritual needs: a rejoinder. Advances: Journal of Mind–Body Health 9(4): 82–84

Aldrich D 1996 Is there evidence for spiritual healing? Advances: Journal of Mind–Body Health 9(4): 4–21

Aldrich D 1996 Notes on the phenomenon of "becoming healthy": body, identity, and lifestyle. Advances 12(1): 51–58

Bergquist S, King J 1994 Parish nursing — a conceptual framework. Journal of Holistic Nursing 12(2): 155–170

Brittain J H 1986 Theological foundations for spiritual care. Journal of Religion and Health 25(2): 107–121

Butcher H K 1996 A unitary field pattern portrait of dispiritedness in later life. Visions: Journal of Rogerian Nursing 4(1): 41–58

Byrd R C 1988 Positive therapeutic effects of intercessory prayer in a coronary care unit population. Southern Medical Journal 81: 826–829

Capra F 1996 The web of life: a new scientific understanding of living systems. Anchor Books, New York

Carson V B, Green H 1992 Spiritual well-being: a predictor of hardiness in patients with acquired immunodeficiency syndrome. Journal of Professional Nursing 8(4): 209–220

Chatterjee I 1989 The concept of spirituality. Allied Pub, Ahmedabad, India

Conwill W L 1986 Chronic pain conceptualization and religious interpretation. Journal of Religion and Health 25(1): 46–50

Coward D D 1990 The lived experience of self-transcendence in women with advanced breast cancer. Nursing Science Quarterly 3: 162–169

Coward D D 1991 Self-transcendence and emotional well-being in women with advanced breast cancer. Oncology Nursing Forum 18(5): 857–863

Davis R 1989 My journey into Alzheimer's disease. Tyndale, Wheaton, IL

Elkins D N 1995 Psychotherapy and spirituality: toward a theory of the soul. Journal of Humanistic Psychology 35(2): 78–98

Elkins D N, Hedstrom L J, Hughes L L et al (1988) Toward a humanistic-phenomenological spirituality: definition, description, measurement. Journal of Humanistic Psychology 28(4): 5–18

Ellison C W 1983 Spiritual well-being: conceptualization and measurement. Journal of Psychology and Theology 11(4): 330–340

Emblen J D, Halstead L 1993 Spiritual needs and interventions: comparing the views of patients, nurses, and chaplains. Clinical Nurse Specialist 7(4): 175–182

Eyre R 1997 Spiritual serendipity: cultivating and celebrating the art of the unexpected. Simon & Schuster, New York

Fehring R J, Miller J F, Shaw C 1997 Spiritual well-being, religiosity, hope, depression, and other mood states in elderly people coping with cancer. Oncology Nursing Forum 24(4): 663–671

Ferder F 1982 Spirituality as personal integration: wholeness and holiness. In: Eigo F (ed) Dimensions of contemporary spirituality. Villanova Press, Villanova, pp 117–142

Fox N J 1994 Postmodernism, sociology, and health. University of Toronto Press, Buffalo, New York

Goddard N 1995a The fourth dimension: conceptualization of spirituality. Unpublished Master's Thesis, University of Edmonton, Alberta

Goddard N C 1995b Spirituality as "integrative energy": a philosophical analysis as requisite precursor to holistic nursing practice. Journal of Advanced Nursing 22: 808–815

Griffin D R 1997 Parapsychology, philosophy, and spirituality: a postmodern exploration. State University of New York Press, Albany

Hall B A 1997 Spirituality in terminal illness: an alternative view of theory. Journal of Holistic Nursing 15(1): 82–86

Helminiak D A 1996 The human core of spirituality: mind as psyche and spirit. State University of New York Press, New York

Hillman J 1975 Re-visioning psychology. Harper & Row, New York

Hilsman G J 1997 The place of spirituality in managed care. Health Progress 78(1): 43–47

Horgan J 1996 The end of science. Addison-Wesley, New York

Idler E L, Kasl S V 1992 Religion, disability, depression and the timing of death. American Journal of Sociology 97: 1052–1079

Kaye J, Robinson K M 1994 Spirituality among caregivers. IMAGE: Journal of Nursing Scholarship 26(3): 218–221

Koenig H G 1993 Trends in geriatric psychiatry relevant to pastoral counselors. Journal of Religion and Health 32(2): 131–151

Koenig H G 1994 Aging and God: Spiritual pathways to mental health in midlife and later years. Haworth Pastoral Press, New York

Koenig H G, George L K, Siegler I C 1988 The use of religion and other emotion-regulating coping strategies among older adults. Gerontologist 28(3): 303–310

Koenig H G, Cohen H J, Blazer D G, Pieper C 1992 Religious coping and depression among elderly, hospitalized medically ill men. American Journal of Psychiatry 149(12): 1693–1700

Koenig H G, Cohen H J, Blazer D G, Kudler H S 1995 Religious coping and cognitive symptoms of depression in elderly medical patients. Psychosomatics 36(4): 369–375

Kraus N, Van Tran T 1989 Stress and religious involvement among older Blacks. Journal of Gerontology: Social Sciences 44(1): S4–S13

Landis B J 1996 Uncertainty, spiritual well-being, and psychosocial adjustment to chronic illness. Issues in Mental Health Nursing 17(3): 217–231

Levin J S 1996 How prayer heals: a theoretical model. Alternative Therapies 2(1): 66–73

Levin J S, Chatters L M, Taylor R J 1995 Religious effects on health status and life satisfaction among Black Americans. Journal of Gerontology: Social Sciences 50B(3): S154–S163

Low J F 1997 Religious orientation and pain management. American Journal of Occupational Therapy 51(3): 215–219

McFadden S H 1996 Religion, spirituality, and aging. In: Birren JE (ed) Handbook of the psychology of aging, 4th edn. Academic Press, New York, pp 162–177

Melton J G 1988 History of the new age movement. In: Basil R (ed) Not necessarily the New Age: critical essays. Prometheus, Buffalo, NY, pp 35–53

Michello J A 1988 Spirituality and emotional determinants of health. Journal of Religion and Health 27(1): 62–70

Mickley J R, Soeken K, Belcher A 1992 Spiritual well-being, religiousness, and hope among women with cancer. IMAGE: Journal of Nursing Scholarship 24(4): 267–272

Miller J F 1985 Assessment of loneliness and spiritual well-being in chronically ill and healthy adults. Journal of Professional Nursing 1(2): 79–85

Miller W R 1997 Spiritual aspects of addictions treatment and research. Mind/Body Medicine 2(1): 37–43

Moberg D O 1997 Religion and aging. In: Ferraro KF (ed) Gerontology: perspectives and issues, 2nd edn. Springer, New York, pp 193–220

Morris L E H 1996 A spiritual well-being model: use with older women who experience depression. Issues in Mental Health Nursing 17(5): 439–455

Muldoon M H, King I N 1991 A spirituality for the long haul: response to chronic illness. Journal of Religion and Health 30(2): 99–108

Murphy M 1992 The future of the body: explorations into the further evolution of human nature. Tarcher, New York

Murphy N 1997 Anglo-American postmodernity: philosophical reflection on science, religion, ethics. Harper Collins, Boulder, Co

Musick M A 1996 Religion and subjective health among black and white elders. Journal of Health and Social Behavior 37: 221–237

Nee W 1968 The spiritual man. Christian Fellowship Publisher, New York

Newman M 1995 Health as expanding consciousness, 2nd edn. National League for Nursing, New York

Olafson F A 1995 What is a human being? A Heideggarian view. Cambridge University Press, New York

Oxman T E, Freeman D H, Manheimer E D 1995 Lack of social participation or religious strength and comfort as risk factors after cardiac surgery in the elderly. Psychosomatic Medicine 57: 5–15

Pargament K I, Ensing D S, Falgout K, Olsen H 1990 God help me: religious coping efforts as predictors of the outcomes to significant life events. American Journal of Community Psychology 18(6): 793–824

Phillips J 1996 Inquiry into the paranormal. Nursing Science Quarterly 9(3): 89–91

Picard C 1997 Embodied soul: the focus of nursing praxis. Journal of Holistic Nursing 15(1): 41–53

Pollner M 1989 Divine relations, social relations, and well-being. Journal of Health and Social Behavior 30: 92–104

Post S G 1997 Ethical aspects of religion in health care. Mind/Body Medicine 2(1): 44–48

Potts R G 1996 Spirituality and the experience of cancer in an African-American community. Journal of Psychosocial Oncology 14(1): 1–19

Pressman P, Lyons J S, Larson D B, Strain J J 1990 Religious belief, depression, and ambulation status in elderly women with broken hips. American Journal of Psychiatry 147(6): 758–760

Reed E S 1997 From soul to mind. Yale University Press, New Haven, CT

Reed P G 1986a Death perspectives and temporal variables in terminally ill and healthy adults. Death Studies 10: 443–454

Reed P G 1986b Religiousness among terminally ill and healthy adults. Research in Nursing and Health 9: 35–42

Reed P G 1987 Spirituality and well-being in terminally ill hospitalized adults. Research in Nursing and Health 10: 335–344

Reed P G 1989 Mental health of older adults. Western Journal of Nursing Research 11(2): 143–163

Reed P G 1991a Preferences for spiritually related nursing interventions among terminally ill and nonterminally ill hospitalized adults and well adults. Applied Nursing Research 4(3): 122–128

Reed P G 1991b Spirituality and mental health of older adults. Family and
    Community Health 14(2): 14–25
Reed P G 1992 An emerging paradigm for the investigation of spirituality in
    nursing. Research in Nursing and Health 15: 349–347
Reed P G 1995 A treatise on nursing knowledge development for the 21st
    century: beyond postmodernism. Advances in Nursing Science 17(3): 70–84
Restak R M 1989 The brain, depression, and the immune system. Journal of
    Clinical Psychiatry 50(2): 23–25
Rogers M 1980 The science of unitary human beings. In: Riehl JP, Roy C (eds)
    Conceptual models for nursing practice, 2nd edn. Appleton-Century-Crofts,
    New York, pp 329–337
Saudia T L, Kinney M R, Brown K C, Young-Ward L 1991 Health locus of
    control and helpfulness of prayer. Heart & Lung: Journal of Critical Care
    20(1): 60–65
Sloan D 1992 Does spirit matter? Advances: Journal of Body–Mind Health 8(1):
    33–39
Smith S W 1995 Power and spirituality in polio survivors: a study based on
    Rogers' science. Nursing Science Quarterly 8(3): 133–139
Sodestrom K E, Martinson I M 1987 Patients' spiritual coping strategies: a study
    of nurse and patient perspectives. Oncology Nursing Forum 14(2): 41–46
Takacs D 1996 The idea of biodiversity: philosophies of paradise. Johns Hopkins
    Press, Chicago, IL
Thomas S 1989 Spirituality: an essential dimension in the treatment of
    hypertension. Holistic Nursing Practice 3(3): 47–55
Wright S D, Pratt C C, Schmall V L 1985 Spiritual support for caregivers of
    dementia patients. Journal of Religion and Health 24(1): 31–38
Wyatt G, Friedman, L L 1996 Long-term female cancer survivors: quality of life
    issues and clinical implications. Cancer Nursing 19(1): 1–7
Wykle M, Segal M 1991 A comparison of Black and White family caregivers'
    experience with dementia. Journal of National Black Nurses Association 5(1):
    29–41
Young C, Reed P G 1995 Elders' perceptions of the role of group psychotherapy
    in fostering self-transcendence. Archives in Psychiatric Nursing 9(6): 338–347

Faith as the 'space between'

Michael Jacobs

INTRODUCTION

Trying to make sense of life is a human preoccupation, and no more so than when someone is taken ill. The search for meaning in life's complexity and in the world we experience is part of the human journey, and it requires of us ways of constructing reality that are helpful and dependable. Inevitably what this suggests, from a psychological perspective at least, is the necessity of belief (a sense of meaning) and faith (the capacity to believe).

Faith provides an intermediate area, a space between, which protects, permeates and filters, contacts, and prepares us for change, as we move throughout life from one way of constructing reality to another. It helps make sense of the relationship between ourselves and our internal and external worlds. As such it is a universal phenomenon, not confined to or by religious creeds nor indeed to obvious spiritual experiences.

What follows is an attempt to map out a psychology of belief. In doing so, I am suggesting that psychology has its part to play in the dialogue about spirituality and health that is represented in this book, and that this link often goes unexamined. I also hope that it may go some way in helping us to understand better one of the ways in which people face illness, and therefore how we might care for them.

ILLUSION OR DELUSION?

In an article on the use of the theory of faith development in pastoral care, two American hospital chaplains (Baldridge & Gleason 1978) illustrate the need for sensitivity to different expressions of faith and meaning. They include an example of a 67-year-old widow undergoing surgery for the removal of her gall bladder. By a grim coincidence, in the next operating theatre surgeons are operating to try and save the life of her grandson, seriously injured in an accident. The grandson dies, adding to a list of deaths the widow has experienced over the last twelve years: another grandson, her husband, her mother and most recently her son. As the chaplain spoke with her about the news of the latest fatality, she said, 'I guess I was supposed to go through these things. ... 'The Lord has seen me through. I've been through a lot in my life, and I bet I can go through a lot more'.

Those who have taken a counselling course might want to suggest the widow shows complete denial of grief and anger. Some people, including in this case the hospital chaplain, might find it intellectually impossible to accept her justification for her stoicism. Others might see in her a good example of Freud's view that religious belief is an illusion: Freud describes 'the benevolent rule of a divine Providence' as an illusion to allay 'our fear of the dangers of life' (1927). In *The Future of an Illusion*, he writes: 'We call a belief an illusion when a wish-fulfillment is a prominent factor in its motivation, and in doing so we disregard its relations to reality, just as the illusion itself sets no store by verification'. In fact he applies his scepticism as much to his own psychological conviction as he does to religion: 'I know how difficult it is to avoid illusions; perhaps the hopes I have confessed to are of an illusory nature too' (1927). This sentence gives some weight to the possibility that Freud's concept of illusion can be extended beyond religion and beyond his own discipline, to other intellectual disciplines.

A different gloss on the widow's response might be found by understanding illusion more positively, as in the writing of the British psychoanalyst D.W. Winnicott. Not only does he say that the capacity for illusion is essential in infant development, but that it lies at the heart of art and religion. What Winnicott suggests (and he admits that we do not yet know how far this is true) is that the world is created anew by every new baby, who starts on that task from birth. The way this world is created depends upon the quality and timing of the mothering. The mother acts psychologically not only as a container, but also as a type of permeable membrane, enabling the baby to relate and come to terms with subjective awareness and increasing exposure to external reality. She is a type of 'space between' the external and the internal worlds of the baby. In time, she introduces her baby to other objects, such as a cuddly toy, a soft blanket, a piece of muslin, or a dummy, any of which can become 'transitional objects' for the baby, serving a similar illusory purpose of adapting to the external environment. The illusion of *possessing* the breast gives way to a more objective perception of the breast, that mother is not the baby's possession. Just as the mother has helped create an illusion in the first place, she also enables this disillusionment to take place. Well-managed disillusionment can lead to new creative illusions. What the mother does for her baby may be replicated (without in any way infantilizing patients) by those in the health professions who offer a listening ear to a person's struggle with the experience of pain and illness.

The difference between Freud and Winnicott (which is an essential one for understanding the living illusions of faith, fantasy and forms of thinking) is that Winnicott does not hold that illusions in adult life are to be viewed negatively. He extends the concept of illusion beyond infancy into the whole of life. The task of weaning is lifelong; it 'continues as one of the tasks of parents and educators' (and, we might also add, of anyone who offers care and counsel). Winnicott (1975) writes:

In other words, this matter of illusion is one which belongs inherently to human beings and which no individual finally solves for himself or herself, although a *theoretical* understanding of it may provide a *theoretical* solution. … The task of reality-acceptance is never completed … that no human being is free from the strain of relating inner and outer reality … relief from this strain is provided by an intermediate area of experience which is not challenged (arts, religion, etc.).

Whatever varieties of faith there may be (whether religious or other belief systems), 'we see through a glass, darkly' (1 Corinthians 13:12). Illusion is a way of constructing experience, and of relating to notions of reality, as well as to the inner world. Winnicott says, 'transitional phenomena are healthy and universal' (1975), and others affirm this, such as the American psychoanalyst, Ana-Maria Rizzuto (1979), who writes:

Men cannot be men without illusions. The type of illusion we select — science, religion or something else — reveals our personal history: the transitional space each of us has created between his objects and himself to find a 'resting place' to live in.

What I believe myself (and if it is my own illusion it serves me well enough that I do not want yet to give it up) is that none of these illusions or ways of believing is right, and none is wrong. If the concept of illusion is to have any meaning it has to be understood as indicating that no one way of believing is more objectively real than any other, even though some forms of belief appear to be more psychologically healthy than others.

Faith, then, is a form of illusion; forms of faith are types of illusion, various or changing attempts to make sense of reality.

Faith is not reality itself, however real it may feel to some people. Faith is an example of Winnicott's phrase 'the space between' — in which we try to make sense of the relationship between us and our internal and external worlds. Because this is a universal phenomenon, spiritual care is relevant to everyone, even if in some contexts or to some people the word 'spiritual' would be the wrong metaphor to use.

FORMS OF FAITH

As Baldridge and Gleason acknowledge in their article (1978), pastoral care and counselling must take account of the different forms which faith takes, the various ways in which beliefs are expressed, and the distinct psychological attitudes that accompany them. These forms cut right across different faiths, different denominations, and even differences between theists, agnostics, and non-theists. This is not simply a religious issue. It is a psychological issue, for therapists as well as pastors. There are, I suggest, clearly identifiable forms of illusion through which people perceive meaning, and by which they live their lives, which are common to many types of thought and discourse, and must be acknowledged if care is to be relevant. There are, for example, fundamentalist Methodists, Muslims, and Marxists; there are countless people who hold magical views about both religion *and* science; and there are universalist thinkers who may be Protestants, Parsees or poets.

These forms, which I describe more extensively in *Living Illusions* (Jacobs 1993), seem to cluster around four themes, which are in themselves metaphors. With some people, spiritual care means accepting their fixed, even rigid, way of believing as sufficient for that person even if not to the taste of the carer. In others, beliefs develop over a period of time, with perhaps a personal crisis, leading to disillusion with the old form, but the creation of a new form of illusion. The carer may have to acknowledge that what a person believes is their way of making sense of reality, even if it is not to the carer's way of understanding. The carer in some situations may be able to assist development to take place, so that a person struggling with an outmoded, unhelpful form of belief, is able to move some way towards one that is more satisfying. In our caring practice, as in life, we must be prepared to look for the different facets which I here describe, although inevitably (since they are not, strictly speaking, stages) at different times, in a different order, and over different issues.

THE FIRST MODE: FAITH AS TRUST AND DEPENDENCY

Belief starts with the primary relationship of mother and baby, and in its first mode has much in common with that early relationship. It is typified by the widow, who has lost so many people close to her, and yet believes in a good God. Her belief system is one that I cannot intellectually accept, but her way of believing is both enviable and profound. It is a state of complete trust in and dependency upon her God. She does not ask questions, does not apportion blame, and does not wallow in guilt. There is a simplicity about her faith in a caring, protecting and nurturing God.

In its finest form (although there is a dark side to it in terms of primitive terror and 'bad magic') this early expression of faith can be imaginative, spontaneous, free, playful, immediate, intuitive, and illogical. It is in one sense *pre-thinking*. It asks no questions. It see no contradictions, such as how such a good God can allow the widow's suffering. This literal and undeveloped faith sometimes gives expression to an apparently mature psychological attitude to existential problems, such as one might expect of a more complex psychological position. This type of illusion is indeed often able to contain anxiety, and appears not to feel anxious about the 'space between', which is safely occupied by simple trust in the whole. People who live with this illusion appear to have little need for explanation, proof or the quest for truth. It is possible, however, that suffering may be one crisis which deals a severe blow to these more straightforward ways of believing, and that people begin to ask questions of meaning and to look for answers.

We do not have to look far for symbols and images to confirm the view of the writers on psychological development that there may be a link between such an unquestioning faith and early infancy. There are strong elements in all religions that are drawn from maternal and nurturing images and symbols. God is described as the provider and sustainer of life: feeding and comforting are characteristic features of the divine. In different religious traditions, communion with the divine and with other worshippers takes place through the act of feeding. This symbolism is particularly profound within the Christian tradition and ritual of the Eucharist. The traditional symbol for Corpus Christi is the female pelican suckling her young from the blood drawn from her own breast; the parallel to a human mother's breast is plain enough; and probably one of the most psychologically powerful phrases in the whole of Christian liturgy is 'This is my Body'. Feeding in caring situations may also be functional, not just religious, and in such acts of feeding care and trust may be built.

James Fowler (1981) in his model of faith development identifies as Stage 1 a time that is filled with fantasy, when a child grasps the world of experience intuitively, with unrestrained imagination and uninhibited by logical thought as adults understand it. In many respects, it is a delightful stage, when everything and anything can be believed. It is the images that capture the imagination, and not any specific message that an adult might wish to attach to them. It is a stage which William James called 'blooming, buzzing confusion'! Fairy stories, and certain religious stories, may help the child's belief that good wins over bad. Such stories often end with what Tolkien calls a 'eucatastrophe', in which everything is turned over for *good* (Tolkien 1964). Some people will want to find a silver lining even in the bleakest hour, looking for some way of turning everything to the good. Where this is a sincere and deep expression of faith it only does damage for the carer to try to undermine it.

What may appear to many helpers as a somewhat idealized form of faith can also have a flip side, which is psychologically much less healthy: it is seen in a person's terror or their fear of 'bad magic'. The danger in this mode of belief is that a child's, or even an adult's, imagination, especially if it is fuelled by illness and pain, can become possessed by unrestrained and uncorrected images of terror and destructiveness. Some forms of religion may exploit that imagination, reinforcing taboos and moral and doctrinal obligations with images of punishment, the devil, and death.

The theologian Paul Tillich suggests that it is anxiety and doubt that push people from this early form of belief (trust and dependency) into the second form of belief. Here simple dependency shifts to dependence upon authority figures for answers to questions that begin to shake the simple trust typified by the bereaved widow. This may also be a point at which the health professional (without having to be an expert in religious or spiritual matters) can give permission for such questions to be asked. Indeed, the health professional who does not claim to know the answers may be more helpful in this situation, in listening to the questions that must be voiced, than the theologically trained minister who is tempted to offer 'pat' answers.

THE SECOND MODE: FAITH AS AUTHORITY OR AUTONOMY

The second form of belief recognizes a 'space between' and begins to feel anxious about it. Contradictions become apparent, and are experienced as discomforting. Something has to fill the space, and belief takes the form of looking for external authority and answers to do so. The title I give this type of faith is 'authority and autonomy': at its worst it is authoritarian, although at its best it provides the authority of tradition as a foundation for the development of a more autonomous expression of belief.

Baldridge and Gleason (1978) give an example of how this type of faith may be encountered in pastoral care. One afternoon the chaplain's bleep goes, with a call from 'Obs and Gynae', asking him to come and say a prayer with a woman who has been in labour for 18 hours. Everything else has been tried, and now she wants to try the church. The chaplain goes to the labour room, talks briefly with the woman, and then says a prayer asking for God's presence with her. Twenty minutes later she gives birth to a fine healthy baby.

At first this case looks like primitive magic, but what the authors emphasize is that this woman needed the authority represented by the church, when the authority represented by the doctors and midwives had apparently failed. Having received that authoritative healing through prayer, her anxiety was diminished sufficiently for birth to take place more smoothly. Her faith does not dwell in her, as it does with the widow, but has to be applied externally to relieve her anxiety. This is not only typical of much organized religion but, also, I have to say, of many other disciplines, including the faith people put in medicine, where answers are sought, and indeed are found or given, in such a way as to forestall more profound questioning. Such faith can temporarily relieve the anxiety of not knowing, the contradictions of experience, and the tensions between perceptions of the external world and internal reality.

This type of faith bears some resemblance to a period of personal development where there is the need to impose some order upon experience. As a child grows and hears stories, and develops stories in her or his own imagination, he or she is involved in making sense of conflicting and anxiety-provoking experiences. The child turns from the powerful imagery of fantasy to attempts at more rational thinking. In this task, a child recognizes the help that adults can give, since they have skills and knowledge to pass on. They provide an authority, which can encourage a child or a young person in becoming autonomous.

The word that summarizes much of this level of development and type of belief is 'control'. Controlling oneself, controlling experience, controlling ideas and thought, and to some extent controlling one's environment, are all major issues. Autonomy also gives rise to problems of how far other people's control (like parental authority) has to be accepted, and how much it can be questioned. The term 'conventional' can mean 'coming together'. This stage of development can be positive in that sense. There is much to be gained in learning conventions and rules. Growing up involves growing up *into* a family, a community, and a society. In learning any new discipline, it is necessary to learn the rules, the conventions, and the traditional knowledge (if only to avoid re-inventing the wheel), before even considering developing new ways of thinking within any discipline.

The problem with this form of faith is that religious thinking can take the form of definitions and ordered systems, seen in the way beliefs are set out in authoritatively stated and ordered creeds. The passion for order can lead to rationalizing contradictions; for example, the Christian church argued over the Trinitarian formula of three persons in one God, or about the two natures of Christ, wholly man and wholly God. In the health setting it is often the irreconcilable contradiction, which the widow referred to earlier did not trouble over, of how a good God can allow pain and suffering. The problem of 'evil' is also a perennial and insoluble dilemma for those who believe in a personal God.

The wish for order, in churches and in society, also tends toward a hierarchical system of authority (which is also seen, in hospital settings, in a more medical hierarchy). In this mode of belief such 'authorities' can become extremely powerful, whether they are parents or experts (and this includes consultants in particular) or even theories. In caring for people who need strictly ordered answers, the slightest word can be taken as a sign of hope or despair. It can also be difficult in caring for some of those who hold strictly ordered views when they are inflexible in their beliefs. Argument is tempting but is unproductive. Recognition of the relief which such belief systems sometimes bring to anxiety in the face of illness and suffering (even if not to our taste) may help the carer to be more tolerant than the patient appears to be. Only if the faith system appears to be cracking, no longer able to hold the anxiety at bay, might the carer try to see if the person could begin to face some of the daunting questions which can no longer be answered in a traditional way.

Conventions can also lead to unthinking conformity. It is important to recognize that not only do the majority of people in religious groups appear to belong in this category (Fowler 1981, 1987, Reed 1978), but also the majority of those who are not committed to religion, or indeed are critical of it. Many of those whose beliefs are either anti-religious or apparently non-religious often demonstrate just as great a conformity to cultural norms as many of their counterparts in the churches, synagogues, mosques, and temples. Achieving autonomy is much less common than we like to think. If anything, there is more openness to the varieties of experience in the first form of belief than there is in this one. There are frequent examples of rigid beliefs in patients that are not confined to those who express religious views. It is possible that some of those who are seen as the most difficult fall into this category, where, hard though it is to listen to them without exploding at their views, it may be helpful to understand just what anxiety is being masked by their complaining and dogmatic tones.

THE THIRD MODE: COMPETITIVE AND COOPERATIVE FAITH

Given the rigidity and the legalism with which so much organized religion is surrounded, it is not surprising that so many people in Western society are not attracted to it, or drift away from it. There can be, however, a more positive result from such drifting, as in the third form for faith experience, which develops from the need for personal autonomy, and for finding a sense of self, over against established beliefs and groups. It often requires breaking away from established groups or organizations, and may involve time 'in the wilderness', although the essence of a true desert or wilderness experience is that it does not come from our own or any one else's expectations.

The trigger is often a personal crisis of one form or another, and obviously may include serious illness in oneself or someone close. We are impelled into a crisis of faith by circumstances which are almost against our will or better judgement. We find ourselves having to confront everything we had once thought was secure. Such a period provides few answers and initially little or no comfort. Only later does security return; and even when that happens, too long a period of security is perhaps a sign of the need to break away again. It is possible that values and meaning may not change dramatically, and that those tenets which have been accepted tacitly now become more explicit, so that ideas are thought through and no longer accepted simply because others say so. But I suspect that, in addition to this, a person typical of this form of belief shows greater openness to alternative explanations and experiences. Although in the early stage of this form of belief there is sometimes an arrogance over against others' beliefs, later there is a real interest in different expressions of belief. It is for this reason that I use the terms 'competitive' and 'cooperative'. In many cases the need to break away and set out in search of a more authentic self often involves setting oneself up in competition with established beliefs and groups, and finding an identity of one's own, sufficient to resist the pressure of blind conformity. This may necessitate some degree of arrogance and egotistic thinking which needs to be distinguished from the subservience to authority seen in the second form of belief.

Others go through such a period of assessing their values and meaning, that in the end do not change dramatically. But they are accepted or adapted through being thought through and made one's own, rather than accepted simply because others say so. In this they may need to accept the support of another, perhaps a health professional, with whom they wish to talk over their ideas, making them their own. This can be a lonely time, and another's presence (where it is unnecessary to agree or disagree, simply to listen and feed back what is being said) may relieve some of the solitude of finding one's way.

This stage can lead to excessive confidence in the conscious mind and in critical thought. Some people may become just as fixed in this type of faith, not recognizing that life is more complex than is allowed for in their emphasis on clear distinctions and abstract concepts. Fowler's model suggests that when people demonstrate 'conjunctive faith', they begin to acknowledge that there are more aspects to their nature than they have hitherto recognized. One aspect of this involves integrating conscious and unconscious — a complex task, where self-deception is a constant risk.

'Conjunctive faith' includes willingness to suspend reason, at least partially and temporarily. This process means re-acquiring the child's (and acquiring the poet's) ability to suspend belief and disbelief. While there are similarities to the first form of belief, 'the willing suspension of disbelief' — Coleridge's phrase about poetic faith (Coleridge 1983) — is a more conscious act, involving toleration of anxiety. By its translation into new and even deeper dimensions, symbols acquire even greater significance, especially when the symbols are allowed to speak for themselves. There may be a case in pastoral care for making available to patients resources which carry much symbolic meaning, meanings which people can use in their own way. Books, music, pictures, the evocative stimulation of the environment through use of colour and space — all these provide possibilities for people to find their own meanings. There may even be rituals which carry such meaning.

Baldridge and Gleason (1978) give an example of this, when a Baptist chaplain was asked by the parents to baptise their baby which was likely to die within half an hour. Baptists do not usually baptise babies, so he was presented with a real dilemma, especially since the parents did not want the baptism for themselves or their baby, but for their own parents who were dedicated church people and would have been deeply distressed were the baby to have died unbaptised. I find this example rather weak. I can see that both minister and parents willingly suspend disbelief in infant baptism in their care for the faith of their parents, but this smacks too much of collusion with magical thinking. This form of belief has more integrity than that. Had the parents asked for a form of ritual that acknowledged the birth and the dying of their baby, expressed in their own terms, that would be a better example both of this type of faith, and of a valid form of spiritual care towards them.

In this type of faith, Fowler identifies a concern to meet with others and learn from them. It is important to test out one's thinking and beliefs, and to learn from the variety of ideas in a supportive group, where people are encouraged to be individuals and not clones. The most productive groups are not those that are made up of like-minded people, but of individuals with different life experiences and a variety of patterns of belief, who are ready to share their thinking, their feelings and their beliefs, without forcing their own experience upon others. Members recognize that their differences allow each person to gain from the other. Such groups seldom end their meetings with agreements, resolutions or conclusions, but members may leave feeling they have expressed themselves and in the process have also learned from others. Health professionals will recognize this type of open thinking if they are themselves open to it, and can, of course, in these circumstances engage in this type of self-disclosure of their own views, knowing that this will not become a heated argument, nor will it be the exercise of authority, but a mutual sharing of the human predicament.

A FOURTH MODE: LETTING GO OF LANGUAGE

There is a fourth expression of faith in which the concerns of previous modes are extended and caught up into a theme of 'letting go': the realization of finitude, and recognition of the inevitability of death; concern for the oppressed and sacrifice of the self for the sake of the wider community; letting go of projections as essentially limited images and ideas; and passing beyond language to concepts that cannot be adequately expressed in any form. These different aspects are set out more fully in the last chapter of *Living Illusions* (Jacobs 1993). Perhaps this mode is most applicable in the health care setting, with those patients and their families where letting go involves loss and/or death.

Erikson (1965) includes 'renunciation' as one of the strengths of old age. Religion has made much of renunciation too, although sometimes it is an overprotective defence against sexuality and the fulfilment of other personal needs and desires, very different from the Zen principle of 'eat when you are hungry, sleep when you are tired' (Watts 1991). In comparing the hypothetical outcome of successful psychoanalysis with the height of mystical experience, Fingarette (1963) identifies a different form of renunciation that they share: the paradox that, in becoming more self-conscious, both the analysand and the mystic cease to be so concerned about themselves. To different degrees, most of us are 'compulsive, obsessive, acutely self-conscious, focusing ... attention upon our feelings and our perceptions, our theoretical distinctions and logical proofs'. Letting go of the self, Fingarette suggests, does not involve self-negation as such, but being able to let go of a particularly anxious form of self-consciousness. It is this which is involved in the way of enlightenment.

FULL CIRCLE

In the third mode of belief a person moves away from slavish dependency upon narrow interpretations of faith typical of the second mode, so that the imagination is capable of embracing 'all kinds of other ideas and aspirations and hopes, things that are to be loved and worshipped' (Cracknell 1986). When the windows of the mind are opened, there is an inexhaustible treasury of beauty and savagery, wisdom and humour, stimulus and comfort — which some will find in religion, others in art, music or literature, and others in nature or in the scientific quest. These treasures are open to many interpretations.

Yet there is also considerable evidence, especially in the literature of different world faiths, that suggests there are experiences where the language of poetry and metaphor are insufficient, and where the images and symbols of art and science fail. Where language is used, it is only through negation that it is possible to convey this type of illusion. Despite their limitations, words paradoxically prove to be capable of enriching understanding, although it is not the words themselves that convey the actual experience.

This particular aspect of belief is letting go of illusion or, in more prosaic terms, the negation of God, religion, and faith. It is an important, if neglected, part of the Western mystical tradition called the via negativa — the way of negation. It is more fully expressed in Eastern religions than in Western faiths. When a wise man in the *Upanishads* is asked to define God, he is silent; meaning that God is silence. When asked to describe God in words, he says 'Not this, not this' (Mascaró 1965). The via negativa involves emptying the mind of the limitations of language and intellectual knowledge. All language about God is in the negative: God is *not* this and *not* that; even, in the words of the pseudonymous mystic Dionysius, 'God is not God'. This is the ultimate, and most difficult, act of relinquishment, as hard as dying or grief. It appears to be a stage of insight, enlightenment or vision which is typified, as the appropriately unknown English mediaeval mystic puts it, by 'unknowing'. These are matters which are difficult to express, let alone to understand, and people may not feel it is safe to express such thoughts. Or they may not need to. They are content, for the moment, within themselves and should not be interrupted. Perhaps what I am wishing to convey most to those who offer pastoral care and counsel is that there will be times when people try to describe experiences which are beyond any words, and where it is impossible to enter fully unless you happen to have 'been there' yourself. Even then they are intensely private experiences. It might be said to be a stage 'beyond illusions'. Again what matters is both acceptance of a person's experience, and perhaps too some sense of involvement with their own mysteries of meaning and being.

Freud's explanation of the illusion that is religion is that we project onto God experiences, fantasies, and fears primarily related to parents and other significant figures from childhood. People may need to do this, in order to find fuller meaning. Giving up such illusions may also involve letting go their traditional faith language, including any intellectual perceptions about God. The French psychoanalyst Lacan wrote: 'What we have in the discovery of psycho-analysis is an encounter, an essential encounter — a *rendezvous* to which we are always called with a real that eludes us' (quoted in Forrester 1990). The same might be said of the spiritual quest.

CONCLUSION

The experience of being ill can be for many people a time of dependency, anxiety, of learning to deal with new realities, or rationalizing contradictions; for some it involves letting go of life. These are all themes to be found in a psychology of belief, that may enable the carer to understand something of the patient's world and the ways in which some forms of belief, in particular circumstances, may be on the one hand helpful and enriching, or, on the other, anxiety-provoking and diminishing.

In describing the different ways in which people believe, and how these beliefs change, it is important to remember the considerable shortcomings of using any model. People are rarely static, since many variable factors impinge upon them, and features from different stages may be present at any one time. Nor is this chapter a blueprint of faith development, or a systematic basis for spiritual care. A psychology of belief must be used cautiously and creatively.

There seems to be an inevitable paradox in a psychology of belief, for it is attempting to describe the ultimately indescribable with mere words. Like many others, I prefer the security and colour of images, even if I do not thirst after facts. When I was writing the last chapter of *Living Illusions*, I was tempted to gather in as many different expressions of this type of belief, in order to demonstrate the essential unity of diverse patterns of discourse, of intellectual disciplines, of artistic and cultural expression and of faith. I had to stop myself, and ask what was the nature of the *illusion* that I was trying to create. Was I being drawn again into the illusion of primal unity? And why? To make the ending neat and comfortable? What of the final disillusion and dissolution? I thought long and hard about my last sentence, and in the end managed to get it the way it needed to be, there and here: 'Do the complexities of all these levels and experiences of belief make it too simple to say there may be nothing there?' (Jacobs 1993).

REFERENCES

Baldridge W E, Gleason J J 1978 A theological framework for pastoral care. Journal of Pastoral Care (USA) 32(4): 232–238
Coleridge S T (1983) Biographia litereria. In: Engell J Bate W J (eds) Collected works, vol 7: 2. Routledge & Kegan Paul, London
Cracknell K 1986 Towards a new relationship. Epworth Press, Manchester
Erikson E 1965 Childhood and society. Penguin, London
Fingarette H 1963 The self in transformation. Basic Books, New York
Forrester J 1990 The seductions of psychoanalysis. Cambridge University Press, Cambridge

Fowler J W 1981 Stages of faith: the psychology of human development and the quest for meaning. Harper & Row, San Francisco

Fowler J W 1987 Faith development and pastoral care. Fortress Press, London

Freud S 1927 The future of an illusion. Penguin Freud Library, vol 12. Penguin, London

Jacobs M 1993 Living illusions: a psychology of belief. SPCK, London

Mascaró J 1965 The Upanishads. Penguin, London

Reed B 1978 The dynamics of religion. Darton Longman & Todd, London

Rizzuto A-M 1979 The birth of the living God. University of Chicago Press, Chicago

Tolkien J R R 1964 Tree and leaf. Unwin, London

Watts A 1991 The spirit of Zen. Harper Collins, London

Winnicott D W 1975 Collected papers: through paediatrics to psycho-analysis. Hogarth, London

Spirituality and the world faiths

Ian Markham

INTRODUCTION

For many health care professionals, the 'spiritual' simply means asking the hospital chaplain to take an interest in a patient. It is viewed as a small supplementary role. The chaplain provides support, while the doctor provides the treatment. The growing interest in the spiritual dimension of health care is rightly viewed as a challenge to this reductionist attitude. To treat people simply as complicated bundles of atoms is to ignore everything significant and important to them. Those sympathetic to the error of this reductionism have seized on the word 'spirituality' to describe the dimension that conventional medicine frequently ignores.

However, the problem is that it is not clear precisely what is meant by 'spirituality'. Spirituality within a religious tradition looks very different from the way medical practitioners talk about spirituality. In the health care literature, the language of spirituality operates in a very general way. The only element completely clear is that it is opposed to the reductionist tendencies of empirical science. Much of the discussion is semi-philosophical: it is an attack on scientific materialism for ignoring the 'spiritual dimension'. Larry and Lauri Fahlberg are representative:

Evidence of an overriding emphasis on the sensate realm — the turf of the five senses — manifests itself in philosophy as materialism, in science as scientism, in social and behavioural science as behaviourism, and in the popular world as the material triumvirate. ... Although health professionals have the desire to go beyond the sensate realm, they are often frustrated in their efforts, given the pervasive philosophical materialism in both professional and scholarly influences. However, these influences often seem to leave us humanistically destitute and spiritually deprived. (Falhlberg & Fahlberg 1991, pp. 273–274)

The project for the Fahlbergs is to construct an account of spirituality which is not overtly religious: so spirituality becomes, 'that which is involved in contacting the divine within the Self or self — "Self" referring to realms of consciousness well beyond the ego' (Fahlberg & Fahlberg 1991, p. 274).

The Fahlbergs are fairly typical: Pamela Reed defines spirituality as 'the human propensity to find meaning in life through self-transcendence; it is evident in perspectives and behaviours that express a sense of relatedness to a transcendent dimension or to something greater than the self, and may or may not include formal religious participation' (Reed 1991, p. 15). L. Ross takes a similar line: 'the spiritual dimension is described and is interpreted as the need for: meaning, purpose and fulfilment in life; hope/will to live; belief and faith' (Ross 1995, p. 457). In each case, spirituality for the health care professional has three elements: first, it is opposed to a reductionist account of personhood; second, it provides a meaning expressed in certain beliefs and values; and third, it is linked to the transcendent. Now Christians would view this as a recognizable, albeit minimal, understanding of spirituality. So for a Christian, a person is not simply a body, but a mind (or spirit or soul) as well. Life has a meaning because the Christian believes that we live in a universe intended by God. And our reason for existing is to worship the transcendent God who is the source of goodness, love, and beauty. Therefore a Christian will recognize the description of 'spirituality', despite the generalized language. Given that 'spirituality in health care' is primarily an Anglo-American debate, one should not be surprised to find that the concept of 'spirituality' involved in that debate is a secularized version of the Christian account. Despite being a deeply religious culture, for Americans to affirm an overtly Christian account seems to go against the constitutional insistence that Church should be separate from the State; and the British, while still sympathetic to religion, tend to find overt Christian expression almost embarrassing. Thus the health care understanding of 'spirituality' is a secularized version of the Christian understanding of spirituality. However, for those from other religious traditions, such an account seems strange and, often, deeply irreligious.

ALTERNATIVE UNDERSTANDINGS OF SPIRITUALITY

Given the complexity and diversity within every religious tradition, it is only possible to provide, in this short chapter, a brief survey of 'spirituality' as recognized by most orthodox adherents of each tradition as representative. Simplification is inevitable. In every case there are alternative accounts even within each religion. In addition, 'spirituality' is not a term recognized by every religious tradition, although it is true that in most there are certain practices surrounding prayer and meditation that seem to take on the characteristics that can be ascribed to the word 'spirituality'.

Islam: spirituality as extinction of the self

Starting then with Islam. It is perhaps worth noting that in early centuries of Islam's development there was considerable suspicion of much 'self-preoccupation' that seemed to be associated with the 'spiritual quest'. Zimmermann explains, 'For centuries the Arabs held out against the spirituality of the solitary life. Their mission was to rule the world, not to renounce it. "No monkery in Islam", goes a slogan of the period preserved as a saying of the Prophet. "The monasticism of this community is the Holy War"' (Zimmermann 1986, p. 499). Yet despite this suspicion of the monastic life, there always was a strong mystical strand, which is even found in the life of the Prophet. It is true that there were always those Muslims who stressed the reality of God as experienced in the individual's life, but it required the brilliant Islamic scholar Ghazali (d. 1111) to integrate into mainstream Islam the tradition of the Sufis. (Islamic mystics called themselves Sufis, which comes from the Arabic word 'suf' meaning 'white wool', because they followed the example of the Prophet who wore clothing made of white wool.) Ghazali's major work, *The Religious Sciences Revived*, brought together Islamic law and ritual with Sufi mysticism.

Since Ghazali, 'spirituality' has been a recognized element of the Islamic faith. Increasingly, Muslims have stressed the mystical life of the Prophet and, indeed, much of the Qur'an is an eloquent tribute to the Prophet's sense of God. So:

God is the Light of the heavens and the earth; the likeness of His Light is as a niche wherein is a lamp (the lamp in a glass, the glass as it were a glittering star) kindled from a Blessed Tree, an olive that is neither of the East nor of the West whose oil well-nigh would shine, even if no fire touched it; Light upon Light. (Qur'an 24: 35)

However, unlike the health care understanding of 'spirituality', where it is a matter of discovering the self beyond the atoms, for the Muslim 'spirituality' involves the complete extinction of the self in God. Our identity merges with the reality of God.

The reason for this is that the central belief of Islam is the oneness and unity of God. The first pillar — the *Shahadah* — simply states, 'There is no God but God, and Mohammed is his prophet'. Monotheism cannot be compromised, hence the Islamic hostility to the Christian doctrines of the Trinity and Incarnation. For the Sufi, this central belief meant that there is no reality apart from God; it becomes 'the means of integration of the human being in the light of the Oneness which belongs to God alone' (Nasr 1987: 312). For those submitting to God (the literal meaning of Islam), the ultimate state is the extinction of the self in God. As the Qur'an puts it:

> And call not upon another god with God; there is no god save He. All things perish, except His Face. His is the Judgement, and unto Him you shall be returned. (Qur'an 28: 88)

And later:

> All that dwells upon the earth is perishing, yet still abides the Face of thy Lord, majesty, splendid. (Qur'an 55: 26–27)

These verses are responsible for the Sufi doctrine of survival after extinction. Although the self is extinct (i.e. completely dependent on God), it continues to survive as a separate identity. One popular image to make sense of this paradox is the unborn child, both within the mother yet surviving. The baby has no existence apart from the mother (and so in that sense is extinct), yet has a continuing identity. Other Sufis seem to go further in understanding the doctrine and seem to talk about their own identification with God himself. Much depends on what is meant when the Qur'an talks about the 'Face of thy Lord'. Seyyed Hossein Nasr explains,

> On the highest level, the realisation of this Face through "self-effacement" — or annihilation, as the Sufis have called it — means to be already resurrected in God while in this life and to see God "wherever one turns". … Through this self-effacement or annihilation, which represents the highest possibility of the human state, the spiritual masters of Islam came to realise the ultimate meaning of the *Shahadah*, which is not only that God is One but also that He is the only Reality in the absolute sense. … He sees God everywhere. … He already lives in Allah's Sacred Name, having died to his passionate self. (Nasr 1987, p. 322)

If health care professionals are concerned about scientific reductionism, what we have here is a 'spiritual reductionism'. In this strand of Islam, we find the 'spiritual' (i.e. God) is the only reality; and the Muslim aspires to live in that state which involves the extinction of the self.

Judaism: discovering spirituality in the mundane

One might expect the other Abrahamic faith which stresses monotheism, Judaism, to be the same. Although it is true that there is a strand that sounds similar (namely, the doctrine of self-annihilation found in the Hasidic movement), the primary stress in Judaism is on the need to discover the 'spiritual' within the world. Arthur Green writes, 'Life in the presence of God — or the cultivation of a life in the ordinary world bearing the holiness once associated with sacred space and time, with Temple and with holy days — is perhaps as close as one can come to a definition of "spirituality" that is native to the Jewish tradition and indeed faithful to its Semitic roots' (Green 1986: xiii). He goes on to bring out the contrast with Western spiritualities: 'Spirituality in the Western sense, inevitably opposed in some degree to "corporeality" or "worldliness", … is unknown to the religious world view of ancient Israel' (Green 1986: xiv). Although an ascetic — world renouncing — strand did develop, Green correctly emphasises that it is a late and, in some respects, alien arrival.

Biblical spirituality is a very 'this worldly' phenomenon. The presence of God, for much of the Scriptures, is located in a 'tent' (a portable temple) and then in the actual temple built in Jerusalem. God encounters his people in a place:

There I will meet with the people of Israel, and it shall be sanctified by my glory; I will consecrate the tent of meeting and the altar; Aaron also and his sons I will consecrate, to serve me as priests. And I will dwell among the people of Israel, and will be their God. And they shall know that I am the LORD their God, who brought them forth out of the land of Egypt that I might dwell among them; I am the LORD their God. (Exodus 29: 43–46)

This sense of encountering God in a place at a certain time within the world lies at the heart of much Jewish ritual. The obligation to observe 613 commandments (many to do with diet and time) ensures that the spiritual becomes part of normal everyday life. Harold Kushner completely understands why to the non-Jew, food laws seem so pointless. Because 'there is nothing intrinsically wicked about eating pork or lobster, and there is nothing intrinsically moral about eating cheese or chicken instead. But what the Jewish way of life does by imposing rules on our eating, sleeping, and working habits is to take the most common and mundane activities and invest them with deeper meaning, turning every one of them into an occasion for obeying (or disobeying) God' (Kushner 1993: 54). The normal takes on a transcendent significance: it ensures one becomes completely human. Harold Kushner puts it rather well when he writes:

Judaism has the power to save your life from being wasted, from being spent on the trivial … Judaism is a way of making sure that you don't spend your whole life, with its potential for holiness, on eating, sleeping, and paying your bills. It is a guide to investing your life in things that really matter, so that your life will matter. It comes to teach you how to transform pleasure into joy and celebration, how to feel like an extension of God by doing what God does, taking the ordinary and making it holy. (Kushner 1993, pp. 293–294)

This, then, is the heart of Jewish spirituality. It is located in the here and now; it stresses certain dispositions and values. Granted the more 'mystical' elements can be found in abundance, but these are always supplementary to the demands of ritual. Nevertheless before leaving Judaism, two mystical strands warrant a mention. The first arose in the period of the Talmudic Rabbis (100 BCE to 200 CE), and it inspired Jewish communities for about a thousand years. It made imaginative use of the chariot image found in the opening chapters of Ezekiel. As the chariot took Ezekiel to God, so contemplatives could ascend to the heavenly halls. The second strand arose in the 12th century. This is the Kabbalah of Spain and Provence. Here we find an elaborate theology, which gives humanity a central role. Because we are created in the image of God, so every human act has a cosmic impact. As the *Zohar* puts it, 'The impulse from below awakens the impulse from on high'. So virtue enables harmony to flow through the creation; wickedness produces discord in the creation. Note that even here in the elaborate Kabbalistic doctrine, the world continues to matter. Spirituality does not involve a denial of the world but an affirmation of it. In this respect the Kabbalah is typical of the rest of Judaism. Spirituality is the recognition of God through the mundane things of the world.

Already, then, we have found two very contrasting accounts of 'spirituality' in Islam and Judaism. Islam stresses the eradication of the self, while Judaism stresses the realization of spirituality through the use of ritual to spiritualize the normal. Both are fairly far removed from the broad concept of 'spirituality' used in health care literature. As we move to those traditions which emerged out of India, we find an even greater distance. Part of the problem is that the assumptions underpinning Indian society are so completely different. Time, for example, is understood in a radically different way. In Western society, the world had a beginning. Up until the middle of the 19th century, this beginning was only 6000 years ago. And, due to the apocalyptic traditions found in Judaism and inherited by Christianity and Islam, we have traditionally believed that the world will end very soon. Traditionally, Western society has been waiting for

God to step in and bring human history to an end. As our society became more secular, the apocalyptic tendencies adjusted to more 'this-worldly' concerns. In the 1970s and 1980s, we expected the world to end in a nuclear catastrophe; as the Cold War dissipated, it was replaced with the ecological catastrophe. The expectation that the world will end soon runs deep in the Western psyche. In the Indian traditions, however, the world is seen as very different. Much to the horror of 19th century Western missionaries, the view is found that the origins of the world are far back in the mists of time — millions of years ago, and the expectation that the world will continue for millions to come. Running parallel with these different concepts of time, we have contrasting accounts of human destiny. In the West, 'we only live once'; in the East, we have lived before and will live again — many times.

These differences lead to different accounts of spirituality, which once again contrast markedly with the accounts offered in health care journals.

Hinduism: spirituality as the discovery of the real self

When it comes to Hinduism, generalizations are impossible. The word simply implies the religions of India. Within India, spiritual expression takes many forms, ranging from sexual affirmation and ecstatic utterance to temple devotion. My discussion will be very limited; I propose to concentrate on an account of spirituality that is found within the *Upanishads*.

The crucial Western illusion is to imagine that the individual ego is the 'real self'. The human ego, according to the *Upanishads*, is entrapped in the world, preoccupied with trivia, and living for the moment. Krishna Sivaraman writes, 'The religious literature of India, in effect, acclaims with a striking unanimity that the actor who dominates the stage of life is a "person," but in the etymological sense of one wearing a mask, a false self. I, as the person (the first person as grammar sanctifies it), is not the real "I" and much less the immortal spirit which I truly am by essence or affinity behind the veil of my nature,' (Sivaraman 1989: xvii). The entanglement with the world (i.e. the immediate activities of human community) leaves the real self undiscovered. The truth about each person is that our real self — the atman — is part of Brahman, the cosmic self, on which everything depends.

Spirituality, then, does involve a renunciation; the term preferred by Sivaraman is 'worldlessness' (Sivaraman 1993: xvi). 'Worldlessness, then, is not "life-and-world negation" but reflects a spiritual mood and a sense of orientation that includes a positive and a negative disposition. Worldlessness is a disposition to live in the world, singly or as a sufficient "human end", but as a means or medium to life "in God", as a condition of life in the spirit' (Sivaraman 1993: xvi).

Instead of directing one's spirituality up and outward towards a transcendent God, in Hinduism one moves down and inward. One discovers the true nature of oneself and in doing that one discovers Brahman (the cosmic self). The methods by which this is attained vary from tradition to tradition. For many people, they will not be ready to obtain moksha (release) in this life. Perhaps they have insufficient good karma (the moral law of the universe) or insufficient time to train under a master. For such people their main responsibility is to play their part in society. (Traditionally, the caste system meant that for many in society, their role is to serve the rest of society, in the hope that higher castes might be given more opportunity to realize moksha and simply hope for a better opportunity in the next life.) For those influenced by Ramanuja, the heart of spirituality is bhakti (devotion); this is the way of love enabled by God.

However, from a health care perspective, perhaps the most interesting way to moksha (release) is that of yoga. The central idea at the heart of yoga is to perceive reality as it really is. Of the six schools of Indian philosophy, yoga is linked with Samkhya (although not exclusively). In the most authoritative text on yoga, *Yogasutra* (Aphorism of yoga), the task of yoga is to make the mind silent. The problem is the 'fluctuations of consciousness'. The tendency of the mind to judge, decide, evaluate, criticize, and organize leaves it unable to see reality as it really is. Ravi Ravindra explains, 'In order to allow the direct seeing to take place, the mind, which by its very nature attempts to mediate between the object and the subject, has to be quietened. When the mind is totally silent and totally alert, both the real subject and the real object are simultaneously present to it: the seer is there; what is to be seen is there; and the seeing takes place without distortion' (Ravindra 1989, pp. 179–180). As one performs the relevant exercises, so one discovers control. Discernment comes as control is developed.

Most Hindus are very unhappy about the Western discovery of yoga as a means to psychic health. 'Rather, yoga proper assumes psychic health, as it does physical health' (Ravindra 1989: 189). It has a religious purpose: one is discerning the ultimate nature of reality. One is discovering the illusory nature of the 'I' of everyday life and engaging with the 'real self'.

Buddhism: spirituality within the ethical

Buddhism can often make an awkward partner in interfaith discussions. Despite emerging from, and sharing many the assumptions of, Hinduism, it has developed in a very different way. It tends to attract all those who are deeply sceptical about metaphysical beliefs. Jane Compson, a Western convert to Buddhism, finds this element the most attractive, when she writes:

> Christianity seems to be inextricably bound up with metaphysics and objective truth, but it seems to me that Hume, Kant, Nietzsche and Wittgenstein completely undermined metaphysics. ... In contrast, the beauty of Buddhism is its simplicity. You need take nothing on authority, and metaphysical beliefs are not a pre-requisite. The Buddha said that he taught only two things, suffering and the end of suffering. (Compson 1996, p. 148)

It is true that the Four Noble Truths, which are at the heart of the Buddha's discovery, do not mention God or a divine being. Instead we have: first, the truth of suffering; second, the truth of the cause of suffering; third, the truth of the cessation of suffering; and fourth, the eightfold Path.

Suffering does not simply describe actual pain, but rather extends out to all the frustrations of being human. Everything changes: even pleasurable moments are marred by the realization that they will end; and every person is a bundle of anxieties about appearance and status amongst our families, friends, and communities. The solution to this suffering is the cultivation of certain attitudes and dispositions. Heinrich Zimmer explains,

> The craving of nescience, not-knowing-better, is the problem — nothing less and nothing more. Such ignorance is a natural function of the life-process, yet not necessarily ineradicable; no more ineradicable than the innocence of a child. It is simply that we do not know that we are moving in a world of mere conventions and that our feelings, thoughts, and acts are determined by these. We imagine that our ideas about things represent their ultimate reality, and so we are bound by them as by the meshes of a net. They are rooted in our own consciousness and attitudes; mere creations of the mind; conventional, involuntary patterns of seeing things; judging and behaving; yet our ignorance accepts them in every detail, without question, regarding them and their contents as the facts of existence. This — this mistake about the true essence of reality — is the cause of all the sufferings that constitute our lives. (Zimmer 1993, p. 66)

Becoming aware of the transient nature of everything (even the sense of one's own self), one ceases to suffer. If everything is transient, then desire and clinging become inappropriate. One will cease to expect a perfectly stable environment, which will mean that all those inevitable disruptions will cease to concern one.

Spirituality, then, is the cultivation of certain dispositions that integrate this awareness of the transient nature of all things into one's life. These are: Right Ideas (the knowledge of the four noble truths); Right Resolution (a commitment to realize the Noble Path in one's life); Right Speech (the means of communication which should be characterized by wisdom and compassion); Right Behaviour (ensure that the mind is in control in everything you do); Right Vocation (one's occupation should be compatible with one's commitment not to harm others); Right Effort (to ensure that motives, attitudes, and dispositions in the mind are compatible with the actions one is required to express); Right Mindfulness (the ability to see things truthfully); Right Dhyana (the capacity to mediate and concentrate the mind) (Goddard 1966, pp. 646–653).

The heart of Buddhist spirituality is a life lived compatibly with the truth discovered by the Buddha in the Four Noble Truths. In the main it is the cultivation of certain ethical dispositions. In this respect it contrasts very markedly with the forms of spirituality found in other religious traditions. It does not start with an engagement or encounter with a divine, transcendent reality. Although it is true that in Mahayana Buddhism, 'worship' of Bodhisattvas (those about to attain Buddhahood) arose, this was a significant development of the Buddha's original teaching.

Nevertheless, it is necessary to touch on some of the more 'mystical' forms of Buddhism. I shall take two very contrasting examples. The first is 'Pure Land' Buddhism. Here we find a straightforward theology of 'grace' (to use Christian terminology). The Bodhisattva Amitabha (an exceptional Buddha-to-be, who is willing to grant wisdom to those seeking it) will save those who put their trust in him. This is done simply by saying, 'I worship Amitabha'. So:

Amida Buddha (Amitabha) is not far from anyone. His Land of Purity is described as being far away to the West, but it is, also, within the minds of those who earnestly wish to be born there. Those who are born in that Pure Land share in Buddha's boundless life; their hearts are immediately filled with sympathy for all sufferers and go forward to manifest the Buddha's method of salvation. (Derrett 1986, pp. 512–513)

Here devotion and trust seem to be the essential feature of the faith; spirituality in this setting involves a dependence on a spiritual being. For the Pure Land Buddhist, you must simply trust Amitabha; this is not unlike the requirement in the

Reformed tradition of Christianity to simply 'trust Jesus'. Links and similarities can be found in the most unlikely of places. Embedded in this most non-metaphysical of religions, we find a metaphysical spirituality.

The second example is entirely different. Zen Buddhism has become popular in the West, partly because it is so antimetaphysical. In Zen the task is to discipline the mind (or, more accurately, to discover the true state of the mind) through a range of complex exercises. D. T. Suzuki writes, 'This getting into the real nature of one's own mind or soul is the fundamental object of Zen Buddhism. Zen, therefore, is more than meditation and Dhyana a stage on the way to transcendental wisdom in its ordinary sense. The discipline of Zen consists in opening the mental eye in order to look into the very nature of existence' (Suzuki 1993: 119). Suzuki is adamant that Zen is not a philosophy (because that implies that logic is only part of mental activity); it is not a religion (because that assumes something transcendent); it is not meditation (because that assumes an object to meditate upon); instead it is 'to come in touch with the inner workings of our being and to do this in the most direct way possible, without resorting to anything external or superadded' (Suzuki 1993, p. 120).

In amongst the myriad forms of Buddhism that have emerged as the tradition has developed, we find two quite contrasting accounts: one which stresses the transcendent, and another which is completely opposed to the transcendent. But, in general, the mainstream Buddhist account sees spirituality as the cultivation of certain ethical dispositions through meditation.

IMPLICATIONS FOR HEALTH CARE

Our brief survey of four different religious traditions has identified at least four different accounts of spirituality. In Islam, spirituality involves the extinction of the self; in Judaism, it is the perception of the spiritual through the mundane; in Hinduism, spirituality is found within you; and in Buddhism, spirituality is found within the ethical.

Certain religious traditions would have a real problem with the threefold meaning of the word 'spirituality', which I identified at the outset of this chapter and which is being so hotly debated among health care professionals. For a Muslim, the transcendent element is everything: Allah is the only reality into which our self needs to disappear. For a Jew, the transcendent is not central; we remember God as we eat and observe the cycles of the week and year. For a Hindu, searching for God outside oneself is wrong, instead God is within. And for the Buddhist, beliefs are being misused if they become the 'meaning to life'. One uses beliefs (like a raft across a stream), but, like everything, one must be willing to give that up.

The temptation for health care professionals is to try and unite all these different accounts of the spiritual. However, this really is impossible. The fact is that they are not compatible — for example, denial of the transcendent is part of Buddhism, while the transcendent is the only reality within Islam. The other tempting strategy is to search for a common denominator. Unfortunately, there isn't one; and even if there was, it is so bereft of content, that its application to health care is less than clear. From an interfaith perspective, it seems clear that both harmonization and the lowest common denominator approach are unsatisfactory. An alternative is needed.

One strategy which might help is to confront the disagreement. When economists (or historians or physicists or whatever) disagree over the nature of the economy (or the past or black holes or whatever), disagreements are confronted. To try and harmonize away a disagreement would look very odd. Instead you are encouraged to examine three elements; first, the internal coherence of two positions making up the disagreement; second, the evidence on either side; and third, the explanatory power (e.g. the compatibility with other knowledge) of each position. At the end of such an analysis, one might be able to commend one account as preferable to another.

If this attitude is taken to all this diversity surrounding the notion of spirituality, then it opens up many new and different areas. It raises the obvious question whether one or another of these accounts might assist the healing process more effectively. Is there any evidence that a Zen Buddhist copes better with illness than a secular Westerner? In other words, a sensitivity to the different types of disagreement should encourage those working in these areas.

Coupled with the need for the debate about spirituality in health care to grapple with the diversity found across the world faiths, there are also more practical implications. The main need is for health care professionals to become much more sensitive to multiculturalism in the treatment of illness. All too often the treatment of diverse cultures simply involves an acknowledgement that one must pay some regard to the dietary requirements or respect the different conventions surrounding gender. There is much more to cultural sensitivity than this.

Cultural difference operates on many levels. As one can see from these different accounts of spirituality, there are different attitudes towards illness operating. A Muslim who is aware of the sovereignty of Allah in all situations and the obligation to accept the will of Allah will, positively, want to know precisely the extent of the illness yet, negatively, might find it difficult to be angry about the situation. Or a Buddhist who believes that the power of the pain of illness is partly determined by the mental disposition of the patient might find the experience of certain illnesses very distressing. Sensitive treatment should involve an awareness of these different cultural perceptions.

CONCLUSION

From the perspective of the world faiths, this debate about the role for spirituality in health care is very interesting. I have argued that much of the debate is operating with a secularized Christian understanding of spirituality. In the other world faiths, there are alternative accounts of spirituality: in Islam, spirituality involves the extinction of the self; in Judaism, it involves the appreciation of the divine through the mundane; in Hinduism, it involves an awareness of the link between one's real self and the cosmic self; and in Buddhism, spirituality is the cultivation of certain ethical dispositions.

Given that the account of spirituality used in health care discussions is quite different from the account of spirituality found in these four religious traditions, what exactly does this imply? Does it mean that this highly generalized account of 'spirituality' is unhelpful?

These are complex questions. Many specialists in religious spirituality and mysticism are very suspicious of the growing popularity of these concepts not only in health care but also in education. It is often argued that to remove the language of 'spirituality' from the vantage point of a particular tradition is to rob the language of all its value and significance. 'Spirituality', it is argued, involves a whole set of metaphysical assumptions about the nature of life, the significance of humans, and the destiny of all things. It becomes a meaningless slogan once disentangled from this framework.

Although I understand this critique, it ignores one very important feature of the discussion. The dominant tradition within our culture is a scientific materialism, which imagines that all illness can be treated physically. Although religious traditions disagree about much, there is agreement here. A secular, humanist account of reality is mistaken, precisely because it disregards the complexity of reality (i.e. the transcendent or spiritual elements). Although this complexity is described in numerous different ways, that it is complex attracts universal agreement.

To treat people holistically is important. But we need to explicate precisely what this means. The best way forward is to listen to the disagreement and engage it. As we listen to the voice of other religious traditions, the task becomes much harder yet much more exciting.

ACKNOWLEDGEMENTS

I am grateful to Shannon Ledbetter and Liz Ramsey who read earlier drafts of this paper. Their helpful comments and observations enhanced the paper considerably. Anybody interested in getting to grips with the variety of conceptions of spirituality in the world religions should look at the 25-volume 'World Spirituality' series published in the UK by Routledge & Kegan Paul, and in the USA by Crossroad.

REFERENCES

Arberry A J 1964 The Koran. Oxford University Press, Oxford
Compson J 1996 Why Buddhism makes sense. In: Markham I S (ed) A world religions reader. Blackwell, Oxford, pp 148–150
Derrett J D M 1986 Buddhism. In: Jones C, Wainwright G, Yarnold E (eds) The study of spirituality. SPCK, London, pp 510–513
Fahlberg L, Fahlberg L 1991 Exploring spirituality and consciousness with an expanded science: beyond the ego with empiricism, phenomenology, and contemplation. American Journal of Health Promotion 5(4): 273–281
Goddard D 1966 A Buddhist Bible. Beacon, Boston
Green A 1986 Introduction. In: Green A (ed) Jewish spirituality: from the Bible through the Middle Ages. Vol 13 of 'World Spirituality' series. Routledge & Kegan Paul, London.
Kushner H 1993 To life: a celebration of Jewish being and thinking. Little, Brown & Co., London
Nasr S H 1987 God. In: Nasr S H (ed) Islamic spirituality: foundations. Vol 19 of 'World Spirituality' series. Routledge & Kegan Paul, London
Ravindra R 1989 Yoga: the royal path to freedom. In: Sivaraman K (ed) Hindu spirituality: Vedas through Vedanta. Vol 7 of 'World Spirituality' series. Routledge & Kegan Paul, London
Reed P 1991 Spirituality and mental health in older adults: extant knowledge for nursing. Family and Community Health 14(2): 15–25
Ross L 1995 The spiritual dimension: its importance to patients' health, well-being and quality of life and its implications for nursing practice. International Journal of Nursing Studies 32(5): 457–467
Sivaraman K 1989 Introduction. In: Sivaraman K (ed) Hindu spirituality: Vedas through Vedanta. Vol 7 of 'World Spirituality' series. Routledge & Kegan Paul, London

Suzuki D T 1993 The essence of Zen. In: Eastman R (ed) The ways of religion. Oxford University Press, Oxford

Zimmer H 1993 Buddhahood. In: Eastman R (ed) The ways of religion. Oxford University Press, Oxford

Zimmermann F W 1986 Islam. In: Jones C, Wainwright G, Yarnold E (eds) The study of spirituality. SPCK, London, pp 498–503

All quotations from the Hebrew Bible are taken from the Revised Standard Version of the Bible.

Faith and belief: a sociological perspective

Grace Davie
Mark Cobb

INTRODUCTION

The National Health Service (NHS) has always been interested, to some extent, in the faith and beliefs of the patients who come into its hospitals. This interest is expressed to the patient through the customary inquiry of a person's religion when they are admitted to hospital. Alongside sexuality, however, spirituality has never been an easy area of investigation; asking for information about religious allegiance requires a certain sensitivity. Despite such difficulties, responses to this cursory question have often been used as decisive information for the provision of spiritual and religious care to patients at critical moments in their lives, not least at the time of death.

The significance of a person's faith and belief to their health and wellbeing is discussed elsewhere in this book. This chapter aims instead to provide a sociological framework for understanding this relationship. The essence of the chapter can be summarized quite simply. Despite a commonly held assumption — strongly bolstered by unrepresentative voices in the media — that secular attitudes prevail in modern Britain, the sociological evidence reveals that relatively few in the population have opted out of religion altogether or out of some sort of belief; in other words, experiences of the sacred or spiritual remain widespread, notwithstanding a recognized and much talked about decline in religious practice.

If health care is to take account of people's faith and beliefs, it will need to be aware not only of the explicit customs and practices of the different faith communities but also of the more subtle and elusive nature of the sacred and spiritual. This chapter is an attempt to chart something of this precarious domain, drawing upon research and discussions dealt with in greater detail in *Religion in Britain since 1945* (Davie 1994). The chapter will be divided into two sections: the first will look at the facts and figures of religion in modern Britain; the second will reflect on these profiles from a more theoretical perspective.

RELIGION IN MODERN BRITAIN: FACTS AND FIGURES
Communities of faith

Any attempt to describe the faith and beliefs of the majority of people in Britain cannot avoid the historical legacy of a country rooted in the Christian tradition. This is equally true whether we accept or reject the parameters of faith. Unbelief, for example, just as much as belief, reflects and is shaped by the Christian tradition of Britain. In terms of the contemporary situation, however, there is an important methodological issue at stake: in attempting to describe the state of the nation in terms of faith and belief we are dealing with semantics and statistics, and both are liable to misinterpretation. Large-scale studies of belief only measure the most obvious and quantifiable aspects of these phenomena. The real implications of these data for health care — as for so many other things — lie well beneath the surface.

The statistical parameters are none the less important. We discover, for a start, that only 14% (Brierley & Wraight 1995) of the population of Britain now claims membership of a Christian church in an active sense. In contrast, the estimated figures for faith communities (as opposed to active membership) in Britain produce a very different picture (Table 7.1). Or to put this in a different way, nominal allegiance is by far the most prevalent expression of religious attachment in modern Britain; no allegiance is moderately rare, though less so than in many countries of Europe. It cannot be assumed therefore that a person who does not attend a service in the hospital chapel will be without spiritual needs or will not want to see the chaplain. Nominal allegiance is a latent factor in spiritual care — one that can remain unexpressed for many years, only to be mobilized in particular circumstances, not least at the onset of illness or injury.

Table 7.1   Estimated membership of faith communities in Britain

Christians	38 200 000
Muslims	1 200 000
Sikhs	500 000
Hindus	400 000
Jews	300 000
Others	300 000

Source: Brierley & Wraight 1995

There is, of course, some difficulty about the meaning of the term 'membership', for the term means different things for different religious communities, an increasingly pertinent factor given the growing pluralism of Britain's religious life. Membership should, moreover, be distinguished from practice; sometimes the two coincide but not necessarily so. But these caveats aside, it remains abundantly clear that both church membership in an active sense and regular church attendance have become minority pursuits in contemporary Britain, and no amount of semantic debate about the precise meaning of terms can disguise that fact. Membership of the principal Christian denominations has declined sharply in the postwar period and continues to do so as the century comes to an end. The rate of decline is, however, uneven, and some denominations have managed to arrest this trend. The independent churches, for example, have seen rapid growth, which is proportionally considerable, but makes little impact upon the overall statistics.

In terms of statistical patterns, the other-faith communities in Britain are similar to the expanding Christian communities: the proportional growth is considerable but the absolute numbers remain small. There is, however, significant diversity within this category which needs constant recognition, for not all of the groups in question have expanded in the postwar period. The Jewish community, for example, used to be larger than it is. A further point is also important. The other-faith communities in Britain are noticeably more varied than their European counterparts, in that Britain (or to be more precise England) now hosts a sizeable Sikh and Hindu population in addition to a significant Muslim presence. The members of all these communities come in the main from the Indian subcontinent; they reflect the nature of British imperial connections. Former imperial connections have also influenced the Christian presence in modern Britain. The Afro-Caribbean population arrived in this country for the same, largely economic reasons as the Asian communities. It is, however, a population of Christian origin and has led in recent decades to a number of thriving Afro-Caribbean congregations.

The Muslims form the largest minority faith community in Britain. Exact figures are difficult to estimate, but Brierley and Wraight (1995) suggest a figure of 1.2 million for the Islamic community (less for the actively religious population). British Muslims come from a variety of countries, but the largest group undoubtedly originates from the Indian subcontinent, notably Pakistan and Bangladesh. But Asian is not coterminous with

Muslim, nor is the Muslim community necessarily homogeneous. Such diversity can be found in all faith communities: it is a mistake to assume that an individual's religious identity can be surmised from his or her ethnic identity. Not only does this cause insult, such stereotyping may also prevent the provision of appropriate pastoral and spiritual care.

Hindus and Sikhs form the two other-faith communities with appreciable numbers of adherents who have arrived in the postwar period. Most of the Hindus and some Sikhs came to Britain from East Africa; they are, therefore, a twice displaced community. And bearing in mind (following Knott 1988) that migration is always a disruptive experience and that religion, like all other aspects of personal and social life, is changed by it, a very wide range of factors need to be taken into account in our understanding of the nature of the immigrant communities of modern Britain. Each faith community deserves sensitive, careful and individual attention, as much from sociologists as from health care professionals. A *limited* pluralism is probably the best way to describe the faith communities of Britain, a description which recognizes the geographical concentrations of particular minorities, namely Jews, Muslims, Hindus and Sikhs. We do, however, live in a multicultural society, a situation which reflects an increasingly interconnected and mobile world just as much as it reflects the changing nature of the British population.

Diversity of belief can be illustrated, finally, in a whole range of new religious movements, whose reputations often belie their negligible size. At one edge lie the relatively well-established sects (Jehovah's Witnesses, Mormons), difficult to distinguish, sociologically if not theologically, from the smaller Protestant denominations. At the other extreme the human potential movements exist in abundance, themselves difficult to distinguish from the New Age, at least in its 'psycho-spiritual' forms. In between can be found a huge variety of groups, distinct in many ways from the surrounding society, but also from each other. No wonder, therefore, that health care systems have difficulty in distinguishing recognizable groups within such diversity, let alone understanding their individual needs. A hospital Patient Administration System, for example, classifies over forty different categories but many are lost within generalizations such as 'other' or simply overlooked as 'not known'.

Returning to the starting point of a supposedly Christian country, relatively few British people either belong actively to a faith community or attend religious services with any regularity, but few people within the population are actively hostile to religion. For most, if not all, of the British retain some sort of religious belief even if they do not see the need to attend their churches on a regular basis. In essence, Christian nominalism rather than secularism is the prevalent belief, and religious organizations of whatever kind — despite their minority status — continue to be a significant feature of modern British society.

Common religion

Studies of faith and belief are inevitably imprecise areas of discussion, a fact which derives largely from the problems of definition. For if sociologists are agreed that the study of religion in contemporary society should include more than the observations about conventional or institutional practice, they are certainly not agreed about an alternative frame of reference. What should or should not be included within these problematic and imprecise categories? Or to put this in a different way, what is the nature of the God in whom the British are supposed to believe? Is he (or she) necessarily a supernatural being or better described as something within the human personality itself? Such confusion is no less evident in the debates concerning religion and spirituality in health care. A search through literature in health care journals produces constructs of 'God' that range from those associated with a deity and religious systems to a non-theistic life principle that activates and influences the individual (Dyson, Cobb & Forman 1997).

In many respects faith and belief have become matters of personal or private choice in Western society. So long as the expression of your views does not offend anyone else, you can believe whatever you like. On the other hand beliefs are seldom self-generated, nor do they exist in a vacuum; they have both form and content — albeit unorthodox form and content — which are shaped as much by the surrounding culture as by the individual believer. Hence a preference for the term 'common' rather than 'private' religion to describe the less orthodox dimensions of believing in modern Britain. It is also helpful to regard variations in beliefs as points along a continuum, rather than the results of choices among coherent systems, some of which are orthodox and some of which are not.

The evidence for the existence of common religion is persuasive (Davie 1994). At one extreme it includes the tendency of British people to approach the churches for rites of passage. In hospitals this is evident in the request for a chaplain at critical times, regardless of religious practice. A review of emergency baptisms in one particular maternity unit (Salter & Watkinson 1994) identified a range of parental motives when this rite was requested: from those — particularly of the Roman Catholic faith — for whom baptism was essential, to those identified as pragmatists who had no apparent religious faith but who 'saw baptism as a way of ensuring that everything possible was being done to help their sick child'. There was, finally, a group whose motives were less well defined but lay somewhere between the other points of view.

The Christian churches hold a variety of views on who should or should not be baptized. There is, however, a latent cultural tradition of baptising infants which is often invoked at times of crisis, a pastoral request which almost all hospital chaplains are willing to consider. It is, however, a characteristic of the last quarter of the 20th century that a far higher percentage of the population experiences this kind of pastoral contact at the time of a death rather than a birth. The arrangements for funerals offer the most obvious situation where pastoral necessity must be balanced against the needs of a particular faith community; it is one to which hospital chaplains are frequently called to respond.

Interestingly, the Roman Catholic version of common religion provokes a rather different line of discussion. Hornsby-Smith (1991), for example, argues for an additional sociological category. The term 'customary religion' is suggested to cover the sort of beliefs that have at least some relation to the official teaching of the Catholic Church as opposed to the much more inclusive common religion, which, Hornsby-Smith maintains, blurs distinctions between religious belief and what is little more than magic or superstition. How far such customary beliefs are distinguishable in practice from the wider area of superstition or even the remnants of pre-Christian religion would seem to be a crucial question in deciding between these two ways of thinking.

Whether approached from a Protestant or a Catholic point of view, it is clear that the content of common religion has, at one end of the spectrum, some link to Christian teaching. At the other end, common religion is enormously diverse, ranging through a wide assortment of heterodox ideas — healing, the paranormal, fortune telling, fate and destiny, life after death, ghosts, spiritual experiences, prayer and meditation, luck and superstition. Spiritual experiences, for example, are a persistent — if partially hidden — phenomenon in contemporary society. An appreciable number of people in Britain claim to have had a religious or spiritual experience of one kind or another. But by no means all

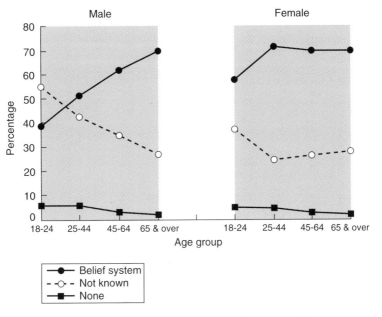

Figure 7.1   Recorded patients' beliefs as a percentage of age group (Hospital Patient Information: 12-month analysis).

of these people are churchgoers, and a significant proportion of those interviewed admitted to hiding such experiences for fear of appearing foolish. An analysis of patients' personal details recorded by a hospital (Fig. 7.1) suggests that substantial numbers of patients are either not being asked about their beliefs or are choosing not to declare them. Therefore, for these patients, their beliefs remain unaccounted for and hidden from view.

Age and gender

Faith and belief cannot be discussed without recognizing at least some of the variables that influence both their form and content. The range, complexity and relationship of such variables should not be underestimated. Regional variations, for example, often related to social and economic differences, produce markedly different religious profiles — a fact which is clearly illustrated in the far from random distribution of other-faith communities in Britain — differences which are reflected in historical, cultural, ethnographic and linguistic factors. The variables of age and gender are rather more straightforward: women, it seems, are almost always more religious than men, as are old people compared with the young, though the figures rise again for children.

In a review of the literature covering the differences between men and women, Walter (1990) takes three dimensions of religiosity: churchgoing, the extent of religious belief, and the content of specific beliefs. It is clear, first of all, that disproportionate numbers of women go to church, although it is important to keep in mind wider demographic shifts in evaluating these data, and particularly the age variable. Older women constitute a group which prospers in modern Britain, demographically speaking, a fact which is likely to skew the churchgoing statistics. It is also the case that women score significantly higher than men on almost any index of religious belief within a questionnaire: the MORI poll of 1989, for example, discovered that 57% of women in their sample believe in life after death, in contrast to 39% of men (Jacobs & Worcester 1990). Within these discrepancies, moreover, Walter is right to emphasize the dimension of private prayer as the one where contrasting behaviours of men and women are at their most marked. Further, if women are asked to describe the God in whom they believe, they concentrate rather more on the God of love, comfort and forgiveness than on the God of power, planning and control. Men, it seems, do the reverse.

Many explanations of these marked variations are offered. Our own inclination, however, is to favour those explanations which underline the proximity of women to birth and death. Understandably, these moments continue — even at the end of the 20th century — to evoke echoes of the sacred, for they must, by their very nature, bring to mind questions about the reasons for existence and about the meaning of life itself. Very few women give birth without any reflection about the mysteries of creation, and very few people watch someone die (especially a close relative) without any thought at all about why that person lived or what might happen to them after death. It is true that medical science has, up to a point, altered the way in which these events are perceived. It is usually the case that birth and death now take place in a medical rather than a domestic environment and both states will be defined in medical parlance. But the giving of birth remains, despite everything, one of the most profound experiences of a woman's life, despite being in hospital at the time. It is equally true that women remain disproportionately involved in the caring roles in our society — in the care of the elderly and dying as well as the nurture of children — even if some of these activities now take place in institutions. Is it all that surprising, in consequence, that the nature of their religiosity is coloured by such experiences?

Older people have always been more religious than the young — a difference which is also indicated in the hospital data (Fig. 7.1). It seems that belief in God, and specifically belief in a personal God, declines with every step down the age scale, as indeed do religious practice, prayer and moral conservatism. Interestingly, however, if the definition of religion is widened to include questions about individual and social health, about the purpose of existence, the future of the planet and the responsibilities of humanity both to fellow humans and to the earth itself, we may find a rather different pattern of 'religious' behaviour among the young. They are, very often, considerably more open to such ideas than their parents.

The data from this section are well illustrated in the following reflections which emerged out of two consultations co-convened at St George's House, Windsor by Paul Avis and Grace Davie in the early 1990s. They concern the experience of a hospital chaplain responsible for the pastoral care of two hospitals in Liverpool, both of which cater exclusively for women. The first admitted patients primarily for gynaecological treatment, including substantial numbers of women in late middle age or even older. The second was the maternity unit for most of Liverpool, admitting mothers for antenatal care and delivery, for the most part women in their late teens, twenties and early thirties. For all practical purposes the constituencies of the two hospitals were similar, apart from the difference in age. Both groups of women were equally pleased to see the chaplain. Indeed in both hospitals there were repeated expressions of gratitude that there was someone in the institution whose business it was to affirm joy, to assuage grief and to comfort in times of tribulation, though the distribution of these tasks might be different depending upon the nature of the hospital. The crucial point, however, from the point of view of this chapter, was the chaplain's awareness that in going about her task in the two hospitals, she had to make different assumptions.

In the first instance, where appreciable numbers of the patients might have had some connection with their churches at least in their youth, the shared vocabulary was evident, if not always articulated: a common language that could be used both in the personal encounter and in the form of worship, even informal worship, that was possible on a Sunday morning. Exactly the same routines in the maternity hospital had, however, to be undertaken rather differently. The younger women were equally appreciative of the chaplain but unable to communicate with her in the same way as their mothers or grandmothers. Similarly, such worship as took place had to be effected without the benefit (or some might say hindrance) of a half-remembered language. Ministry was not necessarily more difficult among the younger women — particularly those emerging from the experience of giving birth — but it had to be approached in a different way. New formulas had to be found for articulating the sacred, for there was nothing to fall back on in this generation of women, born for the most part since 1960.

THEORETICAL REFLECTIONS
Modernity and postmodernity

The background to much that has been discussed in this chapter lies in the shift from an industrial to a postindustrial society, characteristic not only of contemporary Britain, but of much of the Western world in the later decades of the 20th century. The shift is characterized by a variety of features, not least by the pressures brought to bear on both traditional institutions and on widely assumed certainties, in secular as well as in religious life. In contrast, spirituality — of a widely diverse, not necessarily conventional and frequently contradictory nature — shows few signs of diminishing.

Such changes need careful evaluation. Both modern (industrial) and postmodern (postindustrial) societies make heavy demands on most forms of organized religion *but in different ways*. The movement, for example, of large sections of the population away from the countryside to the large centres of population associated with certain kinds of industry was, clearly, disruptive to patterns of religious life established for many centuries all over Europe. It was, moreover, this shift that the classical sociologists observed in considerable detail, a fact which led, among other things, to their generally pessimistic predictions about the future of religion in Western society. Getting on for a century later, however, religious organizations — much reduced, though not always in ways that the classical sociologists had anticipated — find themselves coming to terms with a rather different situation. The larger industrial conurbations, so often the focus of apprehension on the part of the churches, are declining alongside the industries that brought them into existence: so, too, proportionately, are the social class or classes traditionally most reluctant to attend their churches. But the corollary is far from straightforward, for patterns of working-class religion — that is, relatively high levels of belief alongside low levels of practice — instead of disappearing, have become ever more prevalent in contemporary society. So much so that other factors must, surely, be taken into account. One of these concerns the nature of religiosity itself, within which an undeniable evolution has occurred. No longer perceived as duty, religious activity has become, for an increasing proportion of the population, a *leisure* pursuit; one, moreover, which competes for the public's attention alongside all sorts of other pastimes.

A second point requires equal emphasis. Precisely those pressures that have been brought to bear on the religious life of this country are equally present in other dimensions of contemporary society. The NHS itself provides an excellent illustration. It is a public institution which has been forced to undergo profound reforms in response to wider ideological debates as well as to demographic, economic and medical developments (Ranade 1994). Bearing this in mind, it is more accurate to recognize that it is the nature of society which is changing, rather than — or at least just as much as — the nature of faith and belief. Structural pressures brought to bear on the religious sector of society also operate elsewhere. Or to put this in a different way, many of the manifestations of secularization have non-religious rather than religious causes. It is also crucial to recognize that the cultural climate of recent decades has been as hard on secular certainties as it has on religious ones.

Faith and belief — like so many other features of postindustrial or postmodern society — are not so much disappearing as mutating, for the sacred undoubtedly persists and will continue to do so, but in forms that may be very different from those which have gone before. It is within this context that the development of spiritual care within the NHS is taking place. It — like everything else about the NHS — has to adapt to a substantially different society from the one in which it was conceived. But what forms will faith and belief take in Britain as the 20th century gives way to the 21st? In, that is, a society caught up in a changing global economy, but which has a deeply rooted Christian tradition, shared for the most part with its European neighbours, but experienced in a particular and historically definable way. The following section suggests one way of looking at this problem, using the convenient shorthand of 'believing without belonging' as a starting point.

Believing without belonging

It is tempting to see believing without belonging, or the prevalence of unattached religion in contemporary society, as a typical form of postmodern behaviour — one that enables the believer to select at will from the religious goods on offer and to mould these into personal packages that suit a variety of lifestyles and subcultures (the phenomenon known as supermarket religion). Such an assumption seems reasonable enough, given the analysis so far suggested. It becomes, however, a conclusion increasingly difficult to sustain, the harder one looks at the evidence. For in reality believing without belonging rarely represents a consciously selected package. It reflects, rather, a fall-back position acquired by people when they simply do nothing. It becomes, in other words, not so much a choice, but the backdrop against which other decisions are made.

The consequences of such a situation are, however, crucially important for the argument of this chapter, for a lack of attachment to a faith community implies for the great majority of people a lack of discipline in their spiritual orientation. They are, therefore, very much open to the widely diverse forms of the sacred which appear within contemporary society, encouraging rather than discouraging a heterogeneity of belief which includes, in certain circles at least, a number of manifestations of the New Age. One element of religious choice, therefore, seems to mirror the postmodern emphasis on fragmentation, self-selection and self-fulfilment which dominates our culture. In other words it follows, indeed it encourages, the wider trends of contemporary society. But — and once again the qualification is crucial — this is only half the story, for an equally prevalent feature of modern religious behaviour does precisely the reverse. It resists all that is encapsulated in contemporary culture and reasserts, often with great vigour, the traditional certainties, however these are perceived — a reassertion (and the reactive quality is a crucial feature of what is going on) which provides at least one explanation for the undeniable popularity of conservative forms of religion in modern Britain, and indeed in the modern world.

The second of these alternatives is relatively easy to understand. One way of enduring in a fragmented and rapidly changing context (global or otherwise) is to embrace an all-encompassing world view and to live — often in an admirably disciplined way — within this. Or to put this in a different and perhaps more provocative way, the believer not so much rejects fragmentation as takes this to its logical conclusion, selecting one particular fragment of what is on offer and expanding this to form a complete world view. Taken to extremes this tendency results in a series of competing fundamentalisms, a feature of late capitalist development, though one that bewilders many of its commentators. Such fundamentalisms take a variety of forms: some religious, both Christian and non-Christian, and some secular, including within the latter category — to give but two examples — certain types of feminism or radical expressions of regional identity. It is a tendency that every hospital chaplain is likely to encounter at some point.

The sacred and the secular

A final theoretical perspective concerns the elusive links between the sacred and the secular. Contemporary British society is often described as consumerist, an adjective which has a certain ambivalence with respect to the sacred. For there are two possible reactions to this kind of language. The first extends the notion of consumption into the realm of the sacred itself. Not only do we purchase our material requirements, we shop around for our spiritual needs as well. Religious organizations respond to such requests by 'marketing' particular products of an enormously varied nature, some with greater success than others. But alongside the materialism that this is seen to represent can be found a second reaction, one that rejects the notion of consumerism altogether and perceives the sacred in alternative and different forms.

Alternative medicine is an example which displays both these tendencies, not surprisingly since it exists in a bewildering variety of forms. Not only are some of these forms more rather than less compatible with conventional medical practice, they also display very different marketing strategies. But almost all alternative approaches have one feature in common: they attempt to treat the whole person rather than the presenting medical symptoms, whatever these may be. It is, moreover, increasingly recognized that the whole person includes some sort of spirit, together with mind and body. 'Holy' and 'whole' have reacquired their common root; the set-apart or the sacred becomes once more integral to the wellbeing of the individual in question, for no healing can take place while mind, body and soul remain fragmented.

If this is the case at the level of individuals, a rather similar process is taking place with reference to ecological issues, in a debate which evokes profound and difficult questions about the relationship of humanity to the environment. Yet despite the vast difference in scale, the underlying issues are oddly similar to those relating to individual health. For the wellbeing of the planet plainly depends on a right relationship between its various parts. Once the relationship between the parts is disturbed, the health of the whole is inevitably impaired — a point which Jonathon Porritt made in his paper to the 1996 'Body & Soul' conference. A second point follows on: one which renders the conventional divisions between science and religion less and less significant. The experiences of the sacred and the profane can no longer be separated. Indeed in many respects the sacred is no longer contained by conventional boundaries; it is increasingly spilling over into everyday life.

It is within this context that the New Age phenomenon should be placed, for it, too, affirms the continuing significance of the sacred in contemporary society, with its emphasis on wholeness and the spiritual dimension of life. It is true that New Age philosophies are a long way from Christian orthodoxies, and the phenomenon emerges inevitably as an alternative to, even a rival of, conventional religiosity. It is, however, further evidence that the sacred persists in late modern society despite the failure of the mainstream churches to maintain regular contact with the majority of British people (irregular contact remains widespread). The sacred does not disappear, indeed in many ways unconventional forms of religions are becoming more rather than less prevalent in contemporary society. This is, as Beckford (1992) comments, one of the hidden ironies of secularization; it is brought about by diminishing levels of religious control.

CONCLUSION

There are many implications for spiritual care that can be taken from a sociological approach to faith and belief; the most significant is that Britain is far from being a secular society devoid of spiritual experiences and expressions. Whilst it is clear that active membership of orthodox religions has declined, relatively few people subscribe to atheism or abandon religion altogether. This is equally apparent in health care when chaplains are turned to in moments of crisis as people seek to make sense of their lives, often invoking latent beliefs.

A second implication lies in the fact that even if spiritual experiences persist, they often remain hidden and unexpressed. Add to this the realization that patients may well be adversely affected by their illness, disorientation or fear and it follows that exceptional communication skills may be required in dealing with matters of faith and belief in the hospital setting. A cursory inquiry of religious affiliation at the point of admission will almost certainly fail to elicit the more subtle and complex reality that many people experience. Such questions need to be embedded in a far more discursive enquiry, conducted by a person with appropriate skills and training.

The health service, alongside other public institutions, has — quite rightly — made efforts to take account of our multicultural society in seeking to provide a service that is accessible to all in need. Codes of conduct for health care professionals (for example, the UKCC Code of Conduct (see p. 120)) make it quite clear that patients should not be discriminated against on grounds of faith or belief. The Patient's Charter talks of respecting religious and cultural beliefs. This is an area, therefore, that requires great sensitivity and deserves careful attention but which remains susceptible to generalizations, assumptions and stereotypes. It has, for example, already been noted that a person's faith and belief should never be surmised from their ethnic identity, and clearly this applies to white Anglo-Saxons just as much as to any other ethnic community. It is equally necessary to realize that both religious and non-religious categories can mask considerable variations and diversity. Faith communities are seldom completely homogenous; nor, frequently, are those described as atheists as absolute as the term might suggest. The underlying point is nicely illustrated in the following: an elderly patient declaring herself to be 'Jewish' caused much confusion to staff on a hospital ward when she confidently ordered ham sandwiches for lunch.

Health and wellbeing are multidimensional terms that draw upon socioeconomic, environmental and medical models. As the move towards holistic care develops, so too are the spiritual dimensions of health and wellbeing being recognized as part of caring for the whole person. From a sociological perspective, this is a shifting and subtle domain that reflects the wider transformations of late modern society. If health care is to realize its aims, it too will need to respond to the complex challenges of faith and belief which are increasingly apparent in Britain in the late 1990s.

REFERENCES

Beckford J 1992 Religione e società nel Regno Unito. In: La religione degli europei. Edizioni della Fondazione Giovanni Agnelli, Turin, pp 217–289
Brierley P, Wraight H (eds) 1995 UK Christian Handbook 1996/7. Marc Europe, London
Davie G 1994 Religion in Britain since 1945. Blackwell, Oxford

Dyson J, Cobb M, Forman D 1997 The meaning of spirituality: a literature review. Journal of Advanced Nursing 26: 1183–1188

Hornsby-Smith M 1991 Roman Catholic beliefs in England. Cambridge University Press, Cambridge

Jacobs E, Worcester R 1990 We British: Britain under the MORI-scope. Weidenfeld & Nicholson, London

Knott K, 1988 Other major religious traditions. In: Thomas T (ed) The British: their religious beliefs and practices 1800–1986. Routledge, London, pp 158–177

Porritt J 1996 Spiritual values in a secular age, unpublished paper. Body & Soul Conference 1996 Derbyshire Royal Infirmary NHS Trust

Ranade W 1994 A future for the NHS? Health care in the 1990s. Longman, Essex

Salter C, Watkinson M 1994 Emergency baptism on a neonatal unit: first blessing or last rites? Crucible 123–132

Walter A, 1990 Why are most churchgoers women?. Vox Evangelica 20: 73–90

Assessing spiritual needs: an examination of practice

Mark Cobb

INTRODUCTION

In the move to care for the whole person, attention is increasingly being given to the spiritual domain. In an attempt to incorporate spirituality into the overall care of a patient, health care professionals are seeking ways of assessing spiritual needs. Consequently there is a growing interest in methods of assessment to ensure a systematic approach and improve upon what is generally a neglected and arbitrary area of care.

Clinical pathology is the cornerstone of health care, and its diagnostic methods and techniques constitute the benchmark of good clinical practice. However, health is increasingly understood as more than the absence of disease, and ways of understanding how people experience ill health are needed that go beyond disease pathology. If health care seeks to include spirituality in its practice then it will need sensitive ways of identifying spiritual need that are relevant to patients and practicable for health professionals.

DISCERNING NEEDS

It is the basic premise of this book that spirituality is a fundamental characteristic of being human which is affected by the impact of illness, injury and loss. A person's spiritual orientation may be manifest through coherent beliefs and practices or it may be less discernible. Articulating and analysing this dimension is therefore far from easy. It is a diverse phenomenon shaped by the complex patterns of human existence. However, within health care an holistic understanding of the individual is an increasingly tacit assumption and one that underpins much discussion concerning spiritual need. The discovery, or construction (Armstrong 1995), of the whole person has seen a shift in perspective to include social, psychological, and now the spiritual aspects of health, alongside the biological.

The implication is that being human involves a spiritual dimension that is integral to health and significant to illness. It follows that spiritual needs may also arise from that call for assessment and response in the care offered.

Implicit in this argument is a wider debate about what constitutes a healthy person and what it means to be a well human being. Definitions range from the absence of disease to the presence of a 'quality of life', but attempts to be clinically objective inevitably founder on the paradox that, despite powerful diagnostic tools, we cannot distinguish a well person from a sick one. 'Wellness cannot be measured. ... In the final definition, wellness can be distinguished from sickness only by the person involved, sometimes with the help of another person who cares and listens' (Meador 1995). Pathological medicine can search for certain diseases but it struggles to perceive other manifestations of ill health and to recognize the significance of spirituality. Consequently, a patient's spirituality is often unheard and unasked for among the professional community who prescribe treatment and care.

Spirituality often touches upon an individual's greatest fears and aspirations, their thoughts about death and their hopes for life. It is deeply personal, and yet lived out, and something about which many people will readily talk if shown respect and appreciation. It is no wonder that health carers who are poorly acquainted with their own spiritually may easily be embarrassed and feel out of their depth when venturing to speak with others about this. Equally, the ethical framework of trust and confidentiality between health carer and patient does not provide a reason to go beyond a 'need to know' basis of inquiry or the expectation of disclosure.

A lack of calcium can be quantified through a blood test, and the deficit may be redressed by an infusion. Spirituality requires a different form of inquiry that pursues a broader understanding than that provided by physical scientific methods. There are some who suggest that the spiritual should be another diagnostic category and offer definitions of symptoms such as spiritual pain and distress. This, however, also seems a narrow approach to a domain that concerns human biography. Biographies take time to read, they contain peculiarities as well as common themes, history and narrative, revelation and wisdom. Becoming acquainted with another person's spirituality requires more than a knowledge of facts to be systematically processed.

The introduction of markets within the public health system has strengthened a commitment to the voice of patients, their rights and choice, but patients inevitably remain in a disadvantaged and dependent position. A person-centred or patient-focused approach may redress this balance to some extent, but the impersonal methods of science, upon which much of medicine relies, inevitably overlook aspects of our more intimate nature and are insensitive to the spiritual. Discerning and interpreting personal perception and experience in terms of assessing and providing the broader dimensions of health care seems likely to remain something of a poor cousin to pathological medicine. Clearly, spirituality will require some form of exposition and definition if it is to have a place within the health care system and appear other than merely arbitrary and capricious.

The language of need may provide one such route for spirituality, a language accorded considerable weight in health care with its implications for resource allocations. What differentiates a person as being in need is a complex process that takes place between the individual and the wider community. A taxonomy of social need developed by Bradshaw (1972) explored this interaction in terms of

- *normative need*, which exists when an individual or group fall below a standard as defined by experts;
- *felt need*, as perceived and wanted by the individual;
- *expressed need*, as demanded by the individual;
- *comparative need*, which results from studying the equity of a service and identifying gaps in the provision.

When someone is described as being 'in need' it is a permutation of these types of need that exists. In assessing spiritual need, particularly for a given group of people, an exploration of each of these categories is likely to produce useful information that includes the perception of both the individual and the health carer. Thus a picture of need can be built up using the four interrelated criteria.

The model is helpful in separating the many aspects of need that exist in the personal and social context. There are, however, limitations to this model which Bradshaw admits to, not least in the ambiguity and imprecision of the concept of need. However, despite these impediments, health needs assessments are used to inform the strategic planning of health services. To what extent and to what level spiritual care requires such an approach is open to debate, however the dilemma emerges again between the intimate and personal and the corporate and generic. Bradshaw has subsequently reviewed his work in the light of the NHS reforms and critically commented that 'needs assessment has emerged from and quickly settled into the language of priority-setting, economic efficiency, cost-effectiveness and the market-orientated preoccupations of the political right' (1994).

The social policy aspects of health are plainly important determinants in describing a health need, whether that is in terms of NHS strategy or clinical practice. Perhaps what is more fundamental is the understanding of health that is being used. Medical models of health tend to define need in terms of an individual's pathology requiring a cure, whereas social models emphasize health as a resource for living and wellbeing that exists within a wider social context. Health is a condition of human existence and as such it is a basic need, but people require more than an absence of illness to flourish as human beings, and some do so despite their condition. It seems reasonable to suggest that in adopting a social definition of health it can be extended to include spirituality, as indeed it does in palliative medicine.

An alternative approach can be found in models of nursing care which seek to identify the individual needs of the patient. The widely used Roper–Logan–Tierney model borrows from Maslow's theory of human need. Simply stated, Maslow considered that the individual has a positive motivating drive to find fulfilment and strive for goals that make life rewarding and meaningful. At its most basic is the need for survival, higher-level needs include relationships, self-regard and ultimately transcendence. In the Roper–Logan–Tierney model this is approached through the ongoing assessment of the Activities of Living, which include such elements as self-care and sexuality. Spirituality is not referred to explicitly, although the need for worship is included in this model, which is customarily translated as religious practice.

Research into the spiritual needs of patients is not abundant. As an example of a limited study, Emblem and Halstead (1993) interviewed a small sample of surgical patients and compared their views with those of nurses and chaplains. They identified six general categories of spiritual need derived from the interview transcripts:

- religious beliefs and rituals
- values, such as health, acceptance and faith
- relationships
- transcendence of the limits of material existence
- affective feelings, such as peace and comfort
- verbal and non-verbal communication.

By way of comparison the NHS Northern & Yorkshire Chaplains and Pastoral Care Committee (1995) published a document explaining the importance of spiritual care, providing examples of good practice and encouraging health care staff to meet individual spiritual needs. No definition of spiritual need is given, but one is implied in the suggestion that an interview is used to elicit beliefs and values and to consider the patient's wishes concerning:

- worship
- religious health care issues (i.e. areas in which a patient's values or beliefs conflict with care or treatment)
- death, such as customs required before death
- the observance of everyday customs, such as diet and hygiene requirements.

Discerning spiritual needs requires both an openness to the individual patient and the ability to address particular aspects that relate to health care. The more tangible expressions of spirituality, such as rituals and practice, may be more easily dealt with alongside other practical considerations of the patient. However, equally significant spiritual concerns may remain unacknowledged and unexplored.

INTERPERSONAL ASSESSMENT

If spirituality is to be recognized as a dimension of the human experience and a component of health care then some attempt must be made to know what this means for the patient. The traditional question asked of patients upon admission about their religious affiliation may fulfil statistical requirements but it can only provide, at best, a clue to answering the spiritual question. However, before proceeding to obtain a broader picture, it is important to acknowledge the ethical framework within which a patient is asked about their beliefs and experiences, particularly regarding consent and confidentiality. The health care setting, of itself, may suggest to a patient a safe space in which all questions should be answered, but autonomy must be upheld and control over disclosure retained by the patient.

Good communication skills will be fundamental to face-to-face spiritual assessment, and here the principles and practice of counselling are relevant. Lyall (1995) suggests that counselling in the pastoral and spiritual context 'acknowledges the reality of the spiritual experience, and the need of counsellees to make sense of it, either in terms of their present beliefs or by modifying them. But no attempt is made to say *how* that experience is to be interpreted. Rather, the counselling relationship provides the freedom in which clients can make their own interpretations'.

Disclosure of a person's spirituality is seldom spontaneous; it emerges through a relationship of trust, respect and usually out of their life story. Permission must be given and accepted to explore this territory, which may be withdrawn without notice and for many reasons, although it may be reinstated. For some the articulation of spirituality will take place over time, others may deal with it more succinctly, others may communicate it without words, but it is doubtful if any exploration can proceed if the demands upon either person become overbearing or threatening.

It is important that a spiritual assessment is not confined to a predefined structure, but it does need boundaries and it should explore features significant to the health and wellbeing of the patient and their care needs which may include quality of life items. The purpose of the assessment, which should be known by the patient, will determine the level of the discourse and its extent. It is an abuse of the fiduciary relationship between a health care professional and a patient to pursue personal information that is not relevant to their care needs.

An assessment of a patient's spiritual needs will rarely be achieved in a single conversation. Needs are rarely static, and they require regular monitoring and evaluation. Similarly, spiritual care is not an activity to be completed, nor simply an answer to be found. It follows that the assessment of a patient's spiritual needs and the care offered must be incorporated into the overall practice of the care setting, and an integrated discipline among the health care professionals involved. In this way it will be an active and intentional element of care rather than an exceptional practice or a last resort.

The basis of an interpersonal spiritual assessment is the articulation of spirituality through dialogue and mutual exploration. An assessment is not simply seeking to elicit difficulties and problems. There are also positive aspects and therapeutic potential in spirituality which the care team should be aware of and be able to assimilate into the care offered. What is important in the assessment of spiritual need is that serious attention is paid to those aspects of human experience which are often intangible but which affect body and soul, belief and faith, suffering and hope, and the meaning of life, loss and death.

The interpersonal assessment of spiritual needs includes both the subjective and objective, the observed and experienced. The spiritual domain is perhaps a good example of health care as both an art and a science. The science of health care is associated with the tangible objective physical world that can be observed and measured, whereas the art of health care is associated with the subjective intangible world of meanings and value that can only be inferred and alluded to. The two are necessary to deal with the breadth of reality as we know and live it. However, instead of being in a mutual and complementary relationship, the art and science of health care are often viewed antithetically. The distinction here can be epitomized in the dichotomy between quantitative and qualitative methods. 'In the health field — with its strong tradition of biomedical research using conventional, quantitative, and often experimental methods — qualitative research is often criticised for lacking scientific rigour. To label an approach "unscientific" is peculiarly damning in an era when scientific knowledge is generally regarded as the highest form of knowing' (Mays & Pope 1996).

It is apparent that the term 'spiritual need' is open to considerable interpretation because of the breadth of factors that it is intended to cover. It may be shorthand for 'call the chaplain' or it may be a way of expressing the profound despair of a chronically ill patient. In attempting to loosen the association of spirituality with religion and maintain its relevance to health care, spirituality is acquiring new associations. Whilst there are advantages in avoiding a closed definition, there must, however, be a level of general consistency if it is to be of any use. What is at issue here is whether or not the factors which spirituality denotes can attain sufficient definition to be applied to health care without losing an overall sensitivity to this intimate human narrative.

WHAT CAN BE ASSESSED?

Assessment implies a means of evaluation or appraisal that is referenced to a predetermined framework, or at least a notional one, to which can be assigned descriptive nomenclature and some form of order or structure. The more rigorous the assessment the more precise the framework has to be. A passing conversation with someone may elicit enough evidence that the person is 'low in mood', but it would require a far more in-depth discussion to assess whether the person was feeling abandoned by her God. A more rigorous assessment also demands more precise indicators for evaluation that aim to delineate specific attributes or criteria.

A seminal guideline for spiritual assessment was produced by Stoll (1979). This organized system for the collection of data deemed essential in the care of the patient is divided into four areas: the person's concept of God or deity; the person's sources of hope and strength; the significance of religious practices and rituals to the person; and the person's perceived relationship between his or her spiritual beliefs and state of health. The assessment seeks to determine whether the person's God is a helpful and effective resource, what support systems are available, whether or not customs or rituals are important to the person and whether experiences of being ill find an interpretation within the person's belief system. Stoll, however warns that:

The values and beliefs elicited in these areas may or may not be expressed by the person through conventional religious language and rituals. Some people may find these content areas vague, verbally incongruent with their behaviours, or even threatening to discuss. It is important, therefore, to acknowledge each person's right to their own values and beliefs and to respect their right to remain silent about them. (Stoll 1979, p. 1574)

Stoll does not attempt to assign any systematic order of importance to the patient's values and beliefs, although one can be discerned in the guidelines, for example 'without hope, one is left with despair'. Nor is there any attempt to categorize the information in order to indicate spiritual need; this is left to the interpretation of the nurse. By contrast, and in the context of terminal illness, Hay (1989) proposes that spiritual needs can be defined and diagnosed, although he is aware of the linguistic difficulties in spiritual assessment:

Spiritual assessment categories are best thought of as analogous to a third language in service of two others. For example, English spoken by a Spaniard and a German, neither of whom speak the other's language, might facilitate communication, though the nuances of each might be lost. A diagnostic language of spirituality is needed that respects the integrity of psychology and religion, as well as that of non-religious philosophies. (Hay 1989, p. 26)

There is a recognition by Hay that spiritual needs may not be evident until the acuity of suffering can no longer be contained in the physical and psychosocial domains, the consequence being that spiritual needs may not be identifiable separately. However, Hay proposes three categories that are universal to people's spiritual formation: first, that it takes place within a community;

second, that it provides an inner resource for facing life's challenges; and third, that it imparts meaning to reality. This serves as a structure for four diagnostic categories: spiritual suffering, inner resource deficiency, belief system inquiry, and religious needs. Each of these is accompanied by interventions and expected outcomes.

Spiritual suffering, to take one example, is defined as 'inter-personal and/or intra-psychic anguish of unspecified origin' that is characterized by such things as pain, non-compliance with the care plan, guilt and hopelessness. The assessment includes the relationship between interpersonal behaviour and belief system and an exploration of issues such as guilt and remorse. Expected outcomes for this diagnosis involve a reduction in symptoms and behavioural changes, with interventions including the encouragement of reflection upon the relationship between behaviour and the belief system as well as referral to a chaplain.

The spiritual assessment model devised by Hay is intended for use by any member of the care team, given adequate training. It aims to identify problematic areas in the spiritual aspects of a person's life through a structured interview and suggests ways of resolving the problems. The framework of this model has more precision than that of Stoll's with its specific spiritual pathologies, interventions and outcomes. However, both of these assessment methods have a generic approach which may limit their sensitivity and may inadvertently fail to elicit the needs they seek to discern.

In a similar approach to the assessment of individual health care needs, spiritual assessment may benefit from a funnelled approach that begins with a wide-ranging assessment and narrows down to focus on particular concerns. This process can be informed by what we know more generally of people's life and health experiences and any patterns that have been observed. A life cycle framework, for example, recognizes that as an individual passes through time, arbitrary age groups can be established in which there are common key issues such as independence, childbirth or decline (Pickin & St Leger 1993). A faith development model is discussed elsewhere in this book (Ch. 5) which provides psychological indicators of particular issues that may be of concern to those providing spiritual care. What these systematic models provide is a level of coherence informed by common determinants that suggest, at the least, factors which may be considered important in assessing need in particular cases.

The medical specialty of cardiology provides the context for an example of a focused approach to spiritual care. Paterson (1985, p. 249) has suggested that 'for most people, a heart attack comes as a sudden and unexpected encounter with the reality of non-being, an encounter that shatters the groundwork on which everyday existence is built'. Patients in coronary care, simply stated, are not only experiencing loss, both temporary and permanent, but a spiritual crisis involving key issues of faith, meaning, mortality and hope. Spiritual care can be based upon these experiences and focused to offer specific interventions and goals.

A development of this condition-specific model is given by Yim and VandeCreek (1996) in which significant issues are identified for patients preoperatively and at different stages of postoperative recovery. The process begins with a presurgical assessment interview and focuses upon spiritual themes which are relevant to a predetermined model of a thriving recovery, as opposed to a pessimistic recovery by patients. The spiritual assessment is ongoing and attempts to track what is happening with the patient in order to facilitate adjustment and recovery. Spiritual assessment categories include what gives the patient's life meaning, the resources available to the patient to get him or her through the illness, and faith needs. The spiritual assessment is undertaken in conjunction with a more general pastoral assessment that aims to derive a narrative from the patient about his or her experiences of the events, his or her feelings, concerns, cares and how he or she makes sense of what has happened.

These methods of spiritual assessment demonstrate that some form of semi-structured and condition-specific approach may provide a helpful framework to explore issues of spirituality with patients. However, several factors may hinder the process and should be considered.

- Is the assessment practicable for the type of patients being assessed?
- Are the language and concepts used appropriate for all patients?
- Is the health care professional carrying out the assessment capable of dealing with the immediate consequences of what the assessment may evoke?

QUALITY OF LIFE AND WELLBEING

Another approach to spiritual assessment has arisen in the wake of the current interest in the measurement of health-related quality of life. Quality of life in the health care context is frequently cited as an outcome indicator for the efficacy of interventions; however, it is also used as a measure of a patient's perceptions and feelings. It often implies standardized positive and optimum functioning in the physical and psychosocial domains and is proportional to the rating obtained among relevant measurement scales. In health care literature one hypothesis to be found suggests that spirituality is also related to wellbeing. Reed (1992) is representative when she says that 'spirituality is an ever-present, sometimes dominant, part of human experience. As such, it is integral to health — health as defined not necessarily in terms of cure of physical illness but in terms of a sense of wholeness or well-being'.

Taken at first sight there is something absurd in considering that the quality of a person's life, their wellbeing or their spirituality can in some way be rated. And yet we commonly make use of quantitative descriptions in discussing the quality of our own as well as other lives, particularly in pursuing comparisons and in defining a good life. The phrase 'quality of life' has in many ways become popular jargon employed in divergent contexts but with a common appeal. Quality of life and wellbeing are indicators of a preferred ideal, whether they be promoted in the marketing of products or in the pursuit of standards of health. It has been observed therefore that 'quality of life is an amorphous concept, that has a usage across many disciplines. ... It is a vague concept; it is multidimensional and theoretically incorporates all aspects of an individual's life' (Bowling 1995).

Quality of life indicators provide a complementary means of evaluation to clinical pathology, and some are recognizing the significance of domains other than the physical and psychosocial. An oncology research team (Cohen et al 1996) has noted that the physical domain is usually overemphasized in assessing wellbeing in patients of life-threatening illness and that the existential domain is often absent. The McGill Quality of Life Questionnaire (MQOL) was derived from informal patient interviews, a literature review and existing instruments to include physical, psychosocial and existential questions. Existential questions include whether life is meaningful, purposeful and worthwhile and whether it has been a gift or a burden.

The data suggest that MQOL is acceptable, valid and reliable in measuring the quality of life of people with cancer, but the team admits that 'MQOL scores or scores on any questionnaire will never replace the richness of a face to face, in-depth conversation between patient and caregiver' (Cohen et al 1997, p. 17). Self-administered questionnaires are generally considered to produce the best quality data free from the potential bias of an interviewer, but they can only hint at the extensive biography that underpins them.

Patient-based assessments of quality of life generally rely upon predetermined items that are assumed to be relevant to all people in the group being assessed and impose an external set of values on these measures. Inevitably there will be discrepancies between what matters to the assessment (e.g. breathlessness) and what matters to the patient (e.g. attending church). Consequently there has been some attempt to assess what matters to the patient by means of eliciting areas of life judged by them to be most important and to rate their relative and current status. O'Boyle et al (1992) reported that allowing patients to nominate the aspects of their own lives in an evaluation of individual quality of life was more relevant to the patient and applicable across all patients regardless of condition or culture.

Quality of life research is developing and expanding and it raises many useful ideas and questions which can be applied to spiritual assessment. The spiritual domain is a complex phenomenon that does not directly yield quantitative data but is accessible through a qualitative approach with its emphasis on the analysis of experience as interpreted by the individual. This inductive method in general seeks to distil categories and themes from observations in order to extract meaning and develop hypotheses. A number of caveats have already been raised concerning clinical objectivity in spirituality. However, it seems reasonable to assume that in the same way an investigation of the psychological domain may focus upon depression, so the spiritual may focus upon specific components such as hope. Neither is measurable or plainly tangible, but both can be described and assessed indirectly through analogous behaviour.

Portney and Watkins (1993) suggest that intelligence is an example of such a construct. Intelligence can be defined and evaluated using standardized tests like the IQ score. The score is not directly observable, but it is symbolic, referring to the construct of intelligence. In a similar way depression is a construct that cannot be directly assessed, but which can be understood and evaluated. In both these cases, the measurements have to be interpreted, and values placed upon the variables. This is where a level of consensus is necessary if the assessment is to have any general meaning.

The hazards of assessing spiritual constructs are considerable, and there are issues such as bias and cultural sensitivity that need addressing, but there are two important questions that can be asked of an assessment method. First, is it valid: does it measure what it is intended to measure? Second, is it reliable: does it produce consistent results that are free from error? Unfortunately, it can be difficult to determine the strict validity of such an assessment; there is seldom consensus over definitions or even concepts; methodological problems can cause inconsistencies; there may be insensitivity to specific aspects of the construct, and ultimately the uniqueness of individuals suggests items that are incommensurable.

Assessing the impact of illness and treatment on the quality of patients' lives is widening to include spiritual aspects. These may reveal indicators of spiritual need or provide cues for further exploration. What seems important, other than the credibility and recognition that such assessment techniques are gaining, is that they are attempting to access the patient's perceptions and experience. It remains to be demonstrated to what extent spirituality can be captured and assessed in this way.

CONCLUSION

In the drive towards 'evidence-based medicine' and 'quality care' there is an increasing dependency upon diagnostic procedures, standardized routines and clinical audit. These inevitably require needs assessments, measurable outcomes and tangible results in order to manage care and evaluate interventions. All this suggests that if the spiritual dimension is significant to health, and is to be included on the NHS agenda, it may have to demonstrate its worth in ways that conform to a health service focused on efficiency and effectiveness.

This is a dilemma for spiritual care, because as spirituality becomes rationalized and reduced to make it manageable, it begins to lose the subjective and specific human experience which makes it significant. The reason perhaps why there is so much interest in spirituality in health care is because so much has become routine, impersonal and insensitive to the intimate and transcendent realities of life. Assessing spiritual needs will therefore have to balance both empathy and abstraction and the ability to ask questions without providing answers.

Spiritual care can be described without being restricted in definition, and it can be practised in a meaningful way without being confined to routine procedures. As spiritual care becomes more widely recognized, discussed and assimilated there is the danger that its creative and therapeutic potential will become blunted.

REFERENCES

Armstrong D 1995 The problem of the whole-person in holistic medicine. In: Davey B, Alistair G, Seale C (eds) Health and disease: a reader. Open University Press, Buckingham

Bowling A 1995 Measuring Disease, Open University Press, Buckingham, p 2

Bradshaw J R 1972 A taxonomy of social need. In: McLachlan G (ed) Problems and progress in medical care. Oxford University Press, Oxford

Bradshaw J R 1994 The conceptualization and measurement of need: a social policy perspective. In: Popay J, Williams G (eds) Researching the people's health. Routledge, London, ch 3, p 55

Cohen S R, Mount B M, Tomas J J N, Mount L 1996 Existential well-being is an important determinant of quality of life. Cancer 77(3): 576–586

Cohen S R, Mount B M, Bruera E, Provost M, Rowe J, Tong K 1997 Validity of the McGill Quality of Life Questionnaire in the palliative care setting: a multi-centre Canadian study demonstrating the importance of the existential domain. Palliative Medicine 11: 3–20

Emblem J D, Halstead L 1993 Spiritual needs and interventions: comparing the views of patients, nurses and chaplains. Clinical Nurse Specialist 7(4): 175–182

Hay M W 1989 Principles in building spiritual assessment tools. American Journal of Hospice Care, Sept/Oct: 25–31

Lyall D 1995 Counselling in the pastoral and spiritual context. Open University Press, Buckingham, ch 4, p 97

Mays N, Pope C 1996 Rigour and qualitative research. In: Qualitative research in health care. BMJ, London, ch 2, p 10

Meador C K 1995 The last well person. In: Davey B, Alistair G, Seale C (eds) Health and disease: a reader. Open University Press, Buckingham, ch 62, p 424

NHS Northern & Yorkshire Chaplains and Pastoral Care Committee 1995 A framework for spiritual, faith and related pastoral care. The Institute of Nursing at the University of Leeds

O'Boyle C, McGee H, Hickey A, O'Malley K, Joyce C R B 1992 Individual quality of life in patients undergoing hip replacement. The Lancet 339: 1088–1091

Paterson G W 1985 Pastoral care of the coronary patient and family. The Journal of Pastoral Care 39(3): 249–261

Pickin C, St Leger S 1993 Assessing health need using the life cycle framework. Open University Press, Buckingham

Portney L G, Watkins M P 1993 Foundations of clinical research: applications to practice. Appleton & Lange, Connecticut/Prentice Hall, Englewood-Cliffs, N J, ch 2

Reed P G 1992 An emerging paradigm for the investigation of spirituality in nursing. Research in Nursing and Health 15: 349–357

Stoll R I 1979 Guidelines for spiritual assessment. American Journal of Nursing, September: 1574–1577

Yim R J R, VandeCreek L 1996 Unbinding grief and life's losses for thriving recovery after open heart surgery: how pastoral care works in a managed care setting. The Caregiver Journal 12(2): 8–11

The nurse's role in spiritual care

Linda Ross (née Waugh)

INTRODUCTION

A review of the nursing literature shows that spiritual care is part of the nurse's role, though guidelines for its practice are lacking. Within this chapter a conceptual framework for spiritual care is offered, but it has yet to be tested.

Although it would seem that spiritual care is expected of nurses, little is known about their perceptions or practice of that care, the practice of spiritual care itself, or factors influencing its delivery. The results of a major published study addressing these issues are presented and discussed.

The chapter concludes by presenting and discussing the findings of a small pilot study investigating patients' perceptions of their spiritual care needs.

A REVIEW OF THE NURSING LITERATURE ON SPIRITUAL CARE

Definitions of nursing, codes of conduct, models of nursing and guidelines for nurse education show that spiritual care is part of the nurse's role, as discussed below.

Definitions of nursing

Definitions of nursing state that it is the nurse's responsibility to promote and restore health, to prevent illness and to alleviate suffering (Henderson 1977, ICN 1973). For example, Henderson (1977) says that the nurse should:

assist the individual, sick or well, in the performance of those activities contributing to health or its recovery (or to a peaceful death) that he would perform unaided if he had the necessary strength, will or knowledge.

Central to these definitions is the nurse's role in assisting patients to achieve their maximum health potential (Rogers

1970). It has been argued elsewhere that the level of health achieved by an individual will ultimately depend on the extent to which his or her spiritual needs are met (Ross 1995, Waugh 1992). If nurses are to fulfil their function of promoting health, then spiritual care is a nursing responsibility and not an optional extra. It is useful at this point to define spiritual care.

Nursing is a caring profession (Hargreaves 1979) involving itself in helping patients meet needs conducive to health (Henderson 1977). Given this, together with the fact that 'to take care of' has been defined as 'to make necessary arrangements regarding' (Kirkpatrick 1983), spiritual care could be defined as 'to make necessary arrangements for the provision of patients' spiritual needs'.

In addition, a number of nursing authors such as Travelbee (1977) and Henderson (in Henderson & Nite 1978) mention spiritual care explicitly. They acknowledge the need to find meaning in life and suffering. Travelbee (1977) goes further, however, and considers that spiritual suffering, as well as physical or mental suffering, is the concern of the nurse.

Codes of conduct

Both national and international codes of conduct support spiritual care as a nursing responsibility.

The United Kingdom Central Council for Nursing, Midwifery and Health Visiting (UKCC) states that it is the duty of the nurse to: 'Take account of the customs, values and spiritual beliefs of patient/clients' (UKCC 1984a), this being 'a statement to the profession of the primacy of the interests of the patient or client' (UKCC 1984b) which 'places paramount importance upon the interests of patients and clients and the standard of their care' (UKCC 1991). Thus the UKCC acknowledges that spiritual beliefs are of prime importance to the patient and that attention to these should similarly be reflected in nursing practice. The UKCC (1984b) also describes its pronouncement concerning nurses' taking account of patients' spiritual beliefs, to be a 'clear unequivocal statement of the profession's values'. However, rather than being 'clear', this declaration appears rather ambiguous. For instance 'to take account of' could be interpreted in a rather passive way, where the nurse is not actively involved in helping patients meet their spiritual needs. Alternatively, it could be interpreted to mean the nurse's being actively involved in helping patients with these needs. Furthermore, the definition of 'spiritual beliefs' is open to interpretation. For example, it could be viewed in terms of religious beliefs only or in the broader context including the needs for meaning, purpose and fulfillment, hope and so on.

Concerning international codes of conduct, the International Council of Nurses (ICN) (1973), considers its Code for Nurses to be 'a guide for action based on values and needs of society' and states that 'the nurse, in providing care, promotes an environment in which the values, customs and spiritual beliefs of the individual are respected'.

Thus the spiritual beliefs of the individual are recognized and valued by the Council, so much so that this is reflected in its guidelines for nursing practice. However, it is unclear what is actually meant by 'respecting' patients' 'spiritual beliefs' and 'promoting an environment' in which this can be achieved. The fact that the ICN (1977) considers the nurse is 'best able to assess the operating ... beliefs and incorporate her knowledge of them in directing the nursing care' suggests an active rather than a passive role for the nurse in respecting patients' spiritual beliefs. Perhaps this lack of clarity is due to the fact that the Code does not purport to act as a law but rather as a broad guide for practice.

Neither the UKCC nor the ICN could clarify their statements; however, it is worthy of note that the statements concerning patients' spiritual beliefs had been added to the Codes. The UKCC's statement was considered a necessary addition because the Council felt that practitioners often ignore patients' spiritual needs. The ICN added their statement to the Code following its review in 1973.

Codes of conduct acknowledge spiritual care as a necessary and valued part of the nurse's role. Although it is not clear what is actually expected of the nurse, the fact that in both cases additions were made to the Codes reflects the increasing recognition of the influence of the spiritual dimension on health and illness.

Models of nursing

Models of nursing include consideration of the spiritual dimension either directly or by alluding to the individual's wholeness and search for meaning.

Considering those models which do so directly, Henderson (1977) states that it is the duty of the nurse to assist the patient to 'worship according to his faith' and 'practice his religion or conform to his concept of right and wrong'. She interprets spiritual need in the religious context and contends that if religious practice is essential to the individual's sense of wellbeing in health, then it will be all the more necessary during illness. She suggests ways in which the nurse can help patients practise their religion:

- by enabling them to attend a place of worship;
- by contacting and involving appropriate clergy in the patient's care;
- by providing privacy for patient and clergy;
- by making necessary arrangements for them to receive the sacraments.

Watson (in Riehl-Sisca 1989) also includes the spiritual dimension in her model of nursing. Rather than concentrating on the religious aspect, she views spirituality in the broader context of the individual's need for meaning and harmony in existence and for transcendence to a higher level of consciousness. She postulates that if the individual is to experience true wholeness, then he must live in contact with and feed his soul or spirit which is the very core of his being. It is through the soul that the individual can transcend the here and now and coexist simultaneously with the past, present and future, thereby becoming fully integrated and self-actualized. According to Watson, disease or illness can cause or be caused by disharmony in the individual's inner self. The goal of nursing is, therefore, to assist her to achieve inner harmony from which will emanate self-healing. This can be achieved through the 'caring' action of the nurse who is required to be sensitive in order to nurture faith and hope in the patient.

Both Rogers (in Riehl-Sisca 1989) and Weidenbach (in Fitzpatrick & Whall 1983) give consideration to the spiritual dimension by referring to the individual's wholeness, of which the spiritual dimension is part. Fitzpatrick's Rhythm Model (in Fitzpatrick & Whall 1983) includes consideration of the spiritual dimension by concentrating on search for meaning. Other models, such as Roy's Adaptation Model and Neuman's Health Care Systems Model, have been criticized (in Riehl-Sisca 1989) for failing to incorporate the spiritual dimension overtly. Some authors have, therefore, adapted them to include this.

Guidelines for nurse education

Both British and international guidelines for nurse education indicate that spiritual care should be taught to nurses. For instance, in preparation for Project 2000 it was recommended that nurse education should 'provide opportunities to enable the student to … acquire the competencies required to: xiv) identify … spiritual needs of the patient or client, devise a plan of care, contribute to its implementation and evaluation by demonstrating an appreciation of practice and principles of a problem solving approach' (UKCC 1986). This is further reflected in Scotland in the National Board for Scotland's (NBS) consideration of the reforms for basic nurse education. Its aims and objectives include the statement that the nurse will be enabled to 'assess, plan, implement and evaluate care to meet the … spiritual … needs of the individual and family/friends' (NBS 1990). In short, in the UK, nursing students should be taught how to give spiritual care using the nursing process.

On the international scene, the ICN (1973), which, as stated previously, includes spiritual care in its Code for Nurses, considers the code 'will have meaning only if it becomes a living document applied to the realities of human behaviour in a changing society' and that 'In order to achieve its purpose the Code must be … put before and be continuously available to students … throughout their study and work lives'. Furthermore the American Association of Colleges of Nursing (AACN) (1986) recommends that the education of the professional nurse should ensure her ability to 'comprehend the meaning of human spirituality in order to recognize the relationship of beliefs to culture, behaviour, health and healing' and to plan and implement this care.

Having examined definitions of nursing, codes of conduct, models of nursing and guidelines for nurse education, it is evident that spiritual care is within the nurse's remit. However, it would seem that there is a lack of guidelines for the practice of spiritual care, as indicated by the

- lack of a generally agreed definition of 'spiritual';
- lack of literature specifically on spiritual care;
- apparent lack of attention paid to spiritual issues in nurse education programmes;
- lack of research;
- lack of a conceptual or theoretical framework for spiritual care in nursing.

PROPOSED CONCEPTUAL FRAMEWORK FOR SPIRITUAL CARE

If nurses are to be expected to give spiritual care it is important that they have a conceptual framework to guide their practice.

One such framework has been suggested by the author (Fig. 9.1) and is explained below.

An individual entering hospital will do so with particular spiritual needs. Whether or not these needs are met may determine the speed and extent of their recovery and the level of spiritual wellbeing and quality of life they experience. It is important, therefore, that they receive the necessary help to meet their spiritual needs.

One way of ensuring that patients' spiritual needs are met is by using the nursing process as the mechanism to deliver systematic individualized spiritual care (Kratz 1979, Marriner 1983). This will involve identifying the patient's spiritual needs by

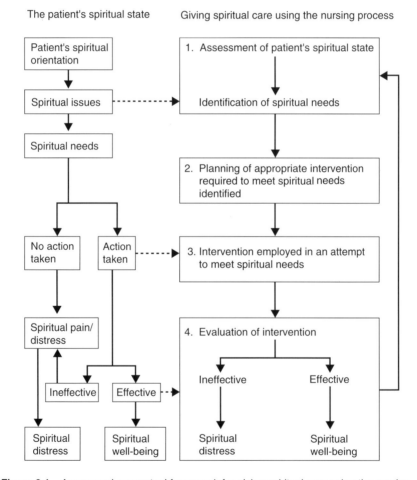

Figure 9.1 A proposed conceptual framework for giving spiritual care using the nursing process (from Ross 1994, with permission).

Box 9.1	Knowledge required for delivery of spiritual care through the nursing process
Stage of nursing process	*Knowledge required*
Assessment	What spiritual needs are. How they can be recognized, i.e. indicators of spiritual distress.
Planning and intervention	What might be appropriate interventions for the meeting of these needs.
Evaluation	What factors would indicate that the needs had been met, i.e. spiritual wellbeing indicators.

conducting a spiritual assessment and, from that, planning and implementing the appropriate interventions to meet those needs and evaluating the extent to which the interventions have been successful. At the outset this seems fairly simple. However, on closer examination, it would appear that in order for each stage of the nursing process to be enacted, it is necessary to have the knowledge identified in Box 9.1, which is currently lacking.

A STUDY OF NURSES' PERCEPTIONS OF SPIRITUAL CARE

Nurses should be giving spiritual care but little is known about how they perceive their role in this, if they practise spiritual care and if they do, how they do it. An exploratory, descriptive study (Ross 1994, Waugh 1992) was, therefore, designed with a twofold purpose:

- to ascertain how nurses perceive spiritual need and spiritual care and to describe how they give spiritual care in practice
- to explore the factors apparently influencing the spiritual care given to patients.

Nurses' perceptions of spiritual need and the provision of spiritual care

A number of questions were posed to answer the above:

- What do nurses understand by spiritual need?
- Do nurses identify patients' spiritual needs?
- How do nurses identify patients' spiritual needs?
- How do nurses respond to patients' spiritual needs?
- Whom do nurses consider to be responsible for responding to patients' spiritual needs?
- How do nurses evaluate the care given?

Staff nurses and charge nurses working full-time day and night duty on 'care of the elderly' wards in National Health Service hospitals in 12 Health Boards within Scotland were selected for the study. Ethical approval was obtained from 12 of the 15 Health Boards, and a purpose-designed questionnaire, containing a mix of open and closed questions, was posted to the population (n=1170) in 1990/91. Using a series of reminder letters, a 67.8% response rate was achieved. Responses were analysed with the help of the Statistical Package for the Social Sciences (SPSS) and the 'Ethnograph'. The results, which follow, are based on 685 usable responses.

What do nurses understand by spiritual need?

Renetzky (1979) defines the spiritual dimension as 'the need to find meaning, purpose and fulfillment in life, suffering and death; the need for hope and a will to live; the need for belief and faith in self, others and God'. The result showed that, as a group, nurses' definitions of spiritual need covered all aspects of Renetzky's definition. Also, the highest proportion of nurses who answered the question (34.1%, n=647) defined spiritual need in terms of the need for belief and faith, this category being predominantly concerned with religious aspects. Other responses included the need for peace and comfort, the need to give and receive love and forgiveness, the need for meaning, purpose and fulfilment and the need for hope and creativity. Overall, though, it would seem that there is a tendency for nurses to view spiritual needs in religious terms.

Do nurses identify patients' spiritual needs?

It would appear that the majority of nurses identified patients' spiritual needs (76.8%, n=655). However, nurses were only asked if they had done so at some point in their practice; therefore, there is no indication of the frequency with which they did this.

How do nurses identify patients' spiritual needs?

Nurses used various indicators in identifying patients' spiritual needs, as shown in Table 9.1. The categories were broken down further revealing that spiritual needs were recognized through non-verbal means of communication in 70% of cases. This suggests that spiritual needs are perhaps more subtle and more difficult to identify than some other needs and that whether or

Table 9.1   Indicators nurses stated they used in recognizing patients' spiritual needs

Indicators	Number and percentage of nurses giving each response (n=685)	
	No.	%
The need was expressed by the patient verbally, e.g. through comments the patient made, or non-verbally, e.g. through facial expression and body language	155	31.4
The need was observed in other ways by the nurse, e.g. by the nurse knowing or sensing	111	22.5
Through distress displayed by the patient, e.g. the patient was awkward, agitated	125	25.3
Through state of helplessness displayed by the patient, e.g. patient was depressed, withdrawn	47	9.5
Through patient's inability to come to terms with situation, e.g. patient displayed regret, guilt	49	9.9
Positive characteristics displayed by the patient, e.g. patient was prepared for death	7	1.4
Did not answer the question	191	

From Ross 1994, with permission

not they are identified may depend on the sensitivity of the nurse.

How do nurses respond to patients' spiritual needs?

Table 9.2 shows that, although some nurses (18.8%) were willing to be intimately involved in helping patients meet their spiritual needs, i.e. those who were prepared to 'be with' the patient, over half (51.6%) were not and chose to refer the patient elsewhere.

Whom do nurses consider responsible for responding to patients' spiritual needs?

Responses showed that almost all nurses answering the question (93.7%, n=660) considered themselves to be responsible, to some extent, for responding to patients' spiritual needs. However, the fact that the majority responded to those needs by referring to someone else suggests that nurses would like to be involved in spiritual care but that this tends not to happen, for whatever reason. 10% of nurses who had identified and responded to a spiritual need (n=495) said retrospectively that they would have responded differently to those needs, and most would have referred the patient to someone else, suggesting that some nurses may feel inadequate about giving spiritual care. It may be that

Table 9.2 Nurses' definitions of spiritual care and/or stated responses to patients' spiritual needs

Definition/response	Number and percentage of nurses giving each response (n=685)	
	No.	%
Recognizing/respecting/meeting patients' spiritual needs	44	6.8
Facilitating participation in religious rituals	43	6.7
Communicating: listening to or talking with	42	6.5
Being with the patient: caring, supporting, showing empathy	121	18.8
Promoting a sense of wellbeing	58	9.0
Referring to other professionals	333	51.6
Expressed difficulty in defining or giving spiritual care	4	0.6
Did not answer the question	40	

From Ross 1994, with permission

some of these nurses consequently feel unable to provide such care themselves.

How do nurses evaluate the care given?

The majority (84.4%) of nurses who evaluated the care they had given (n=500) considered their interventions to have been effective. 463 nurses described the indicators they used in their evaluations, as shown in Table 9.3. The highest proportion (37.6%) concluded that the care they had given was effective because of eustressing (opposite of distressing) characteristics displayed by the patient, e.g. the patient was more calm, relaxed, peaceful. Other nurses reached this conclusion through the patient's confirming that her need had been met, through the nurse's sensing or knowing that the need had been met and by improvements in the patient's mood and acceptance of her situation. Some nurses found it difficult to evaluate the care they had given.

Overall, it would seem that non-verbal cues were used by nurses to evaluate the effectiveness of their care.

Factors which appeared to influence the spiritual care given

Factors which may have influenced the spiritual care nurses gave were identified in two ways: by cross-tabulation and interviews.

Table 9.3   Indicators nurses stated they used in evaluating the effectiveness of responses to patients' spiritual needs

Indicators	Number and percentage of nurses giving each response (n=685)	
	No.	%
Eustressing characteristics displayed by the patient	174	37.6
Patient appeared brighter in mood	48	10.4
Patient's ability to accept situation	35	7.6
Patient confirmed that her need had been met, e.g. by comments, change in attitude	78	16.8
Nurse felt that the need had been met (not necessarily confirmed by the patient), e.g. nurse sensed a change	46	9.9
Nurse felt that the need was not met or not completely met	28	8.0
Nurse expressed difficulty in assessing the effectiveness of his interventions	54	9.7
Did not answer the question	222	

From Ross 1994, with permission

Variables were cross-tabulated, and four were found to be significantly associated with the identification of spiritual needs by nurses. These related to the grade and belief system of the nurse and the type of ward and geographical area in which s/he was working.

Grade. Charge nurses were more likely to identify spiritual needs than were staff nurses; however, this could not be explained by their length of experience or age.

Belief system. Nurses claiming religious affiliation were more likely to identify spiritual needs than those claiming none.

Type of ward. Nurses working on varied wards (e.g. long-term care and geriatric medicine) were more likely to identify spiritual needs than those working on non-varied wards (e.g. long-term care only).

Geographical area. Nurses working in some Health Boards were more likely to identify spiritual needs than those working in others.

These findings raise more questions than they answer.

In order to identify possible reasons for the above associations and to further explore factors which may have influenced the spiritual care nurses gave, semi-structured interviews were conducted with a sample of 12 nurses selected on the basis of set criteria. Although generalizations could not be made and the sample was too small for statistical treatment, it was hoped that the more detailed information would give some clues to possible factors influencing the spiritual care given.

Results of interviews

Analysis of the interviews revealed that four main groups of factors appeared to influence the spiritual care nurses professed to give. These related to the patient, other professionals, the environment and the nurse (Fig. 9.2).

The patient. It seemed that any factors which interfered with nurse–patient communication e.g., deafness, dementia, made it difficult for nurses to identify spiritual needs. Perhaps if there

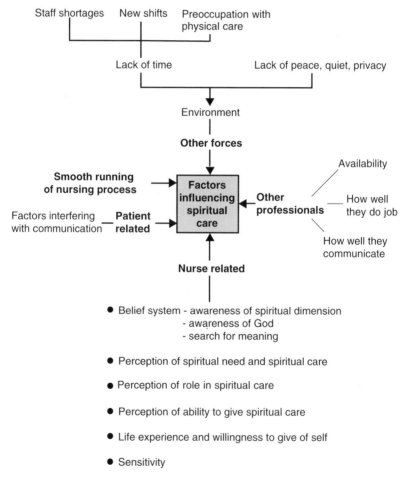

Figure 9.2 Factors, emerging from the qualitative part of the study, which appeared to influence spiritual care (from Ross 1994, with permission).

were a predominance of patients suffering from conditions such as dementia in long-term care wards this could explain the previous finding that nurses employed on non-varied wards reported having identified fewer spiritual needs than those working on varied wards.

Other professionals. Spiritual care was sometimes hindered if clergy were not available, if there was a lack of communication between the two disciplines, or if in the nurse's opinion, they had not performed their job properly. This finding perhaps suggests the need for greater collaboration between nurses and clergy.

Environment. Nurses reported that lack of time, whether because of low staffing levels, preoccupation with physical care or new shift patterns, interfered with the giving of spiritual care. This finding perhaps has implications for administrative decisions. Given the influence of the spiritual dimension on health, perhaps it would be more economically viable in the long term to ensure adequate staffing levels and to alter shift patterns to increase rather than reduce staff overlap. Nurses also reported that a lack of peace, quiet and privacy hindered them from delivering spiritual care. This perhaps has implications for ward layout. It may be beneficial to have a quiet room set aside, without a television, where patients could have peace and quiet or to have a rest hour as part of the ward routine.

The nurse. It appeared that spiritual care could be given on different levels. Some nurses were able to identify a broad range of spiritual needs and respond personally at a deep level. Others could identify a narrow range of needs only and responded at a more superficial level, i.e. by referring to someone else. The way in which nurses gave spiritual care seemed to depend on a number of personal characteristics. Nurses who gave spiritual care at a deep level demonstrated the following characteristics.

- They were aware of the spiritual dimension in their own lives. This finding suggests that the spiritual awareness of the nurse may be more important than the religious label she adopts in determining how she gives spiritual care.
- They had experienced crises which seemed to act as forces for growth, enabling them to become more self-actualized. This suggests that the life experience or maturity factor may be more important than the grade of the nurse in determining the care given by him.
- They were willing to give of themselves at a deep personal level, which may be associated with their own life experience and spiritual awareness.
- They were particularly sensitive, perceptive people.

Nurses who gave spiritual care at a superficial level demonstrated some or all of the above characteristics to a lesser degree.

To summarize, nurses seemed fairly good at assessing patients' spiritual needs and evaluating the care given, but felt less able to respond to those needs, possibly because of feelings of inadequacy. Factors relating to the patient, nurse, other professionals and the environment appeared to influence the delivery of spiritual care, although further research would be required to verify this. It was mentioned at the beginning that there is little British research addressing nurses' views on and practice of spiritual care; similarly there is little research into the patient's perspective.

A PILOT STUDY INVESTIGATING PATIENTS' PERCEPTIONS OF THEIR SPIRITUAL CARE NEEDS

A small pilot study was carried out to test an interview schedule designed to ascertain elderly patients' perceptions of their spiritual needs and care (Ross 1997). Ten (six male and four female) patients from a geriatric assessment ward in one Edinburgh hospital were interviewed in the summer of 1995. Half were married, four widowed and one divorced. Only one was still working, the rest having retired. Most had been admitted with heart problems one to two weeks previously. The results are by no means generalizable but nevertheless give insight into some patients' views of their spiritual needs and care.

Patients' views on spiritual matters

The ten subjects offered thirteen views on spiritual matters. Five thought spiritual things related to religion. Some considered spiritual matters to be broader, including the needs for support, moral standing, peace and meaning. One person was unsure what spiritual things might be and another considered spirituality to be a very private thing.

Seven patients believed in God, six describing their belief in terms of being aware of a God who was looking after them and one as an inability to accept that we cease to exist after death. Four felt their belief had been very helpful to them in coping with life's difficulties, one helpful to some extent, one not much and one not at all helpful.

Patients' experiences of spiritual needs

Of the ten patients, two had experienced spiritual needs at some point in their lives and two had never experienced any spiritual needs. Six said they had experienced spiritual needs since coming into hospital. These patients had been in hospital only a few weeks, raising the possibility that spiritual need may arise during longer hospital stays.

Of the eight patients who claimed to have experienced spiritual needs, half reported having had more than one need. Six reported needs that were religious in nature, such as to pray or attend church. Needs related to making sense of things or finding meaning were reported by some patients. Coming to terms with loss or guilt were mentioned, as was a need to be accepted or have a feeling of love and belonging. Issues around death and dying, life after death, and moral standing were raised. For instance one patient mentioned the need to treat people decently.

Concerning religious needs, although some patients were aware that a church service was held from time to time, none had attended. They either had not been given sufficient information about the location or timing of the services or had been unable to get someone to take them. Several patients mentioned trying to pray at night with their face turned to the wall while pretending to sleep. This raises the issue of the degree of peace, quiet and privacy in the wards. Although six patients felt they had enough peace, quiet and privacy, four felt that these attributes could be increased by reducing the number of people per room and by removing portable televisions from shared rooms. Perhaps prayer and reflection would be easier if a quiet room was provided or if patients were made aware of the chapel's availability.

Four patients reported the need to make sense of or to find meaning in life. None of the patients, however, had talked to anyone about any of their needs. Only two out of the six patients who had experienced spiritual needs since coming into hospital said they would like to speak to someone such as a chaplain about these needs. Perhaps they were reluctant to do so because of their experience to date. Six people had seen a member of the clergy since coming into hospital. Most expressed dissatisfaction with the visit for several reasons: they felt 'jollied along' when they didn't want to be 'jollied along'; they wanted to speak about more serious things than the weather; they did not know it was a member of the clergy until he had gone; the visit was too short. These findings perhaps highlight the importance of clergy's introducing themselves to patients as well as being prepared to broach more serious issues for discussion.

CONCLUSION

A review of the nursing literature shows that spiritual care is expected of nurses, but little is known about how nurses perceive or practise spiritual care. The results of the author's doctoral study revealed that, within the sample, nurses seemed able to identify patients' spiritual needs and evaluate the care given, mainly through observing non-verbal cues displayed by the patient; however they were less willing or able to respond personally to these needs.

Charge nurses claiming religious affiliation and working on varied wards in certain geographical locations seemed most likely to have identified spiritual needs. However, from the limited sample interviewed, it would seem that personal characteristics of the nurse were perhaps more important than these other factors in determining whether the nurses gave spiritual care or not and how they gave it. Further research is required to clarify this.

Furthermore, the availability and performance of other professionals, together with environmental factors and those concerned with nurse–patient communication, appeared to determine if and how nurses gave spiritual care.

From the patient's perspective, the results of a small pilot study revealed that most elderly patients interviewed experienced spiritual needs while in hospital. Enabling them to attend hospital services and providing a quiet room for prayer or reflection are examples of ways in which the elderly might be helped to meet their spiritual needs whilst in hospital. The conclusions that can be drawn from this small study are, however, limited, highlighting the need for further research. Studies conducted on a larger scale which seek to identify the type of help patients would like with their spiritual needs would be helpful in providing nurses and other health care professionals with the necessary guidelines for promoting spiritual health and alleviating spiritual suffering of their patients.

ACKNOWLEDGEMENT

Sections of text on pp. 126–134 adapted from Ross (1994) with permission. Sections of text on pp. 119–125 adapted from Ross

1995 *The spiritual dimension: its importance to patients' health, well-being and quality of life and its implications for nursing practice in the* International Journal of Nursing Studies volume 32 pp. 457–468. Copyright 1995, with kind permission from Elsevier Science Ltd, The Boulevard, Langford Lane, Kidlington OX5 1GB, UK.

REFERENCES

AACN 1986 Essentials of college and university education for professional nursing. AACN, Washington, DC, p 5

Fitzpatrick J J, Whall A L 1983 Conceptual models of nursing: analysis and application. Robert J Brady, New Jersey, p 190

Hargreaves I 1979 Theoretical considerations. In: Kratz C R (ed) The nursing process. Baillière Tindall, London

Henderson V 1977 Basic principles of nursing care. ICN, Geneva, p 4

Henderson V, Nite G (eds) 1978 Principles and practice of nursing. Macmillan, New York

International Council of Nurses (ICN) 1973 Code for nurses: ethical concepts applied to nursing, ICN, Geneva

International Council of Nurses (ICN) 1977 The nurse's dilemma: ethical considerations in nursing practice. ICN, Geneva, pp vii, 14

Kirkpatrick E M (ed) 1983 Chambers 20th Century Dictionary. Chambers, Edinburgh, p 190

Kratz C 1979 The nursing process. Baillière Tindall, London

Marriner A 1983 The nursing process: a scientific approach to nursing care, Mosby, Missouri

NBS 1990 Nursing education: preparation for practice 1992. NBS, Edinburgh, p 16

Renetzky L 1979 The fourth dimension: applications to the social services. In: Moberg D O (ed) Spiritual well-being: sociological perspectives. University Press of America, Washington, pp 215–254

Riehl-Sisca J 1989 Conceptual models for nursing practice, 3rd edn. Appleton & Lange, Connecticut

Rogers M 1970 An introduction to the theoretical basis of nursing. Davis, Philadelphia

Ross L A 1994 Spiritual aspects of nursing. Journal of Advanced Nursing 19: 439–447

Ross L 1995 The spiritual dimension: its importance to patients' health, well-being and quality of life and its implications for nursing practice. International Journal of Nursing Studies 32(5): 457–468

Ross L A 1997 Elderly patients' perceptions of their spiritual needs and care: a pilot study. Journal of Advanced Nursing 26: 710–715

Travelbee J 1977 Interpersonal aspects of nursing. In: Yura H, Walsh M (eds) 1982 Human needs 2 and the nursing process. Appleton Century Crofts, Norwalk

UKCC 1984a Code of professional conduct for the nurse, midwife and health visitor, 2nd edn. UKCC, London, p 2

UKCC 1984b Exercising accountability: a framework to assist nurses, midwives and health visitors to consider ethical aspects of professional practice. UKCC, London, p 4

UKCC 1986 Project 2000: a new preparation for practice. UKCC, London, pp 40–41

UKCC 1991 Code of conduct under review. Register 9: 6, p 6

Waugh L A 1992 Spiritual aspects of nursing: a descriptive study of nurses' perceptions. Unpublished PhD thesis, Queen Margaret College, Edinburgh

Spirituality and the scientific mind: a dilemma for doctors

Margaret Whipp

INTRODUCTION

Over thousands of years of human history, the practice of healing and the profession of religion were bound inextricably together. It is only recently — over a few centuries in our Western world — that the two have diverged sufficiently for George Eliot to remark in *Middlemarch*, 'It is seldom a medical man has true religious views — there is too much pride of intellect'.

In Britain, the history of organized health care goes back to the mediaeval monasteries. Brother herbalists with their *hospices* and *infirmaries* combined spirituality and science in their compassionate service to the sick in need. The Rule of St Benedict insisted that 'the care of the sick is to be given priority over everything else, so that they are indeed served as Christ would be served'. For centuries the gospel texts, 'I was sick, and ye visited me' and 'Inasmuch as ye have done it unto one of the least of these my brethren, ye have done it unto me' were inscribed over the portals of British hospitals, inspiring a whole culture of health care that was deeply grounded in the spirit of Christ.

The dichotomy between body and soul developed slowly. In 1139, monks, nuns and clergy were forbidden to study medicine, whilst Chaucer's somewhat later Doctor of Physic's 'studie was but littel on the Bible'. Church leaders tragically opposed new medical learning. Dissection was outlawed until the 16th century. The church pronounced against Harvey's theory of the circulation of the blood, as it later would oppose anaesthesia, contraception and the application of genetic engineering. The gradual advancement of medical science away from superstition and quackery was not encouraged by conservative religious leaders who feared the autonomy of an increasingly secularized profession. By the time of the Enlightenment, the dominating rationalism of Cartesian philosophy drove theology and medical science finally asunder.

THE WAY SCIENCE WORKS

Science works through a process of logical analysis. Detailed observation, critical experimentation, systematic rationalization and careful verification combine to yield new knowledge of cause and effect. Science can explain what goes wrong with our bodies, and its explanations are expressed in terms of cause and effect. The more complex the system under investigation, the more detailed is the potential explanation of each subsystem and microsystem that contributes to an elaborate chain of mechanistically linked causes and effects. The relentless pursuit of the cause behind each effect leads to specialization, subspecialization, and the inevitable fragmentation of the system in question.

Such an approach is ruthlessly objective. It dissects and dismembers in order to understand, but it cannot reckon with subjectivity, purpose or will. These things are simply beyond the remit of scientific method.

It is this powerful process of science that has shaped the dominant medical model of disease. On this model, the body is a system composed of innumerable mechanisms, which may function or malfunction in any number of scientifically determinable ways. To understand these bodily malfunctions in a way that permits effective intervention is to hold a very powerful key indeed to human health and wellbeing. This is the remarkable power of medical science.

It is by reason of this healing power that the medical model has remained dominant. Effective explanations of infection, biochemistry, malignancy and pathophysiology have enabled enormous strides to be taken in the control of previously lethal disorders. Modern medicine has doubled the life expectancy and enhanced the life quality immeasurably in those societies, mainly in the Western world, where it is widely available.

Yet the medical model has been fiercely criticized (Box 10.1). The scientific paradigm in which it is rooted is inherently reductionist, unable to embrace and reflect the whole breadth of moral and philosophical, social and spiritual perspectives that bear on human health and healing. It is against this background of astonishing efficacy on the one hand, and terrible limitations on the other, that the medical model based on science must be re-evaluated from the perspective of spirituality.

THE CONCERNS OF SPIRITUALITY

Compared with the cool clarities of medical science, our attempts to chart the spiritual dimensions of human life appear

---

Box 10.1 Criticisms of the medical model

1. Individual bias
The medical model tends to isolate the human body from its social context and value. Consequently the diagnosis and management of disease is highly individualistic.

2. Curative bias
The medical model is a problem-solving approach best suited to curable conditions. It has much less to offer in prevention, and is ill-suited to the care of chronic disability, or the response to incurable disease.

3. Physicochemical bias
Many critics question the relevance of the medical model to mental disorders, in which social and personal factors, less amenable to scientific evaluation, are more important than physicochemical derangements.

4. Technological bias
The medical model treats the human body as a malfunctioning machine. Many patients feel threatened and dehumanized by aggressive technical interventions of which they have little understanding or control.

5. Pathological bias
The medical model assumes that *diseases* are real entities which it seeks to overcome. This interpretation is philosophically questionable, and difficult to apply, for example, to genetic disorders, infertility, or physical and mental handicap.

6. Objective bias
By asserting the objective physical basis for disease, the medical model ignores the subjective meaning of sickness for the sufferer, and the moral and spiritual dimensions of the sick person's experience.

7. Professional bias
The medical model rests on a base of detailed knowledge and professional expertise. This casts the patient in the role of an amateur, with little knowledge or power in the doctor–patient relationship.

---

fascinating, yet fearfully imprecise. To the scientifically trained mind, 'spirituality' is a bit like jelly — good if you can grasp it, but notoriously difficult to pin down. 'Spirituality' is not a system or a technique, nor is it an area of objective investigation or verifiable explanation. In none of these ways does 'spirituality' reflect the criteria and tenets of science.

Spirituality is best described as *the human concern for things that matter*. It is a concern for meaning, value and relationship, and the ultimate meaning, value and relationship that are found in God. It is a concern that longs for human fulfilment, and agonizes over every kind of human diminishment. Spirituality, therefore, is profoundly concerned for health, and for all that human wholeness will entail.

In the field of health care, issues of spirituality are never far beneath the surface. Spiritual problems, however difficult to diagnose and define, are recognized by most doctors to contribute significantly to patient distress. Yet these more or less apparent spiritual concerns of patients are not the only manifestations of spirituality in the field of health. From my own research it is clear that spirituality plays a central part in the vocational awareness of doctors, and their attitude to the doctor–patient relationship. And within the wider context of public health, Baroness Macfarlane has charted the spiritual dimensions of our national 'culture of care' (Macfarlane 1995). Spirituality, as a concern about our authentic humanity, is more than a merely private question of individual wellbeing.

Spirituality and patients: syndromes of spiritual distress

Spiritual distress becomes acute when the meaning, value and relationships that secure authentic humanity are seriously threatened. Spiritual distress may coincide with physical or emotional distress, but it manifests a deeper kind of pain, reflecting a different and profoundly disturbing human dis-ease.

The features of spiritual distress have been discussed in other chapters. It is not the purpose of this chapter to re-examine those features, rather to emphasize that typical symptoms can and should be recognized in susceptible patients. The diagnosis of spiritual distress is something that can be learnt and should be taught. Health care professionals need a greater appreciation of the situations that are likely to provoke spiritual distress.

Degradation and dehumanization are the common factors in most of these situations. To illustrate some typical situations in which spiritual concerns become paramount, let us consider four currently prevalent syndromes.

Ostracized by AIDS

For people with HIV, the appalling prognosis of AIDS is matched in dreadfulness only by the cruel stigma that goes with it. AIDS victims are in many ways the lepers of modern society, struggling not only with a destructive and debilitating disease, but also with the moral censure of a self-righteous society, fearful of contamination.

The spiritual questions raised by AIDS — for patients, friends and carers — can be painful in the extreme, and their implications will be considered at length in the following chapter. Their problems represent in a most pointed way the complexity and the challenge of spiritual distress.

Overwhelmed by technology

Despite the many positive contributions of science and technology to human health and happiness, there can be no doubt that these benefits have cast a very long and threatening shadow. From the simple phobic anxiety of the patient who fears being engulfed in the scanner to the highly complex and ethically intractable questions of how we may rightly interfere with the beginnings and endings of life, there is a deeply spiritual dimension to the widespread human fear of technology. We have a deep-seated dread of being overwhelmed by technology at our most tender and vulnerable points of humanity. This horror is summed up in the degrading and dehumanizing expression of 'being treated like a lump of meat'.

Overridden by finance

Closely linked to the rapid growth of technology is the soaring cost of health care provision. Not a week goes by without some report of hospitals running out of money to treat their patients. The once unthinkable notion that some patients are too expensive to be treated is now an everyday opinion. Medical costs and human values seem to be set on a collision course, in which the only brakes being applied are those of constant downward economic pressures. Yet the debate about costs and values is at heart a spiritual debate, in which the central issue is the way we measure human worth. Whilst there are economic insights and financial methods that have to be addressed in any realistic debate, the critical question is how to assert the immeasurable values of human life over material costs. For patients reckoned too expensive to be treated, there can be nothing more dehumanizing that to be simply wiped off the accountant's slate like a bad debt.

Beyond help

Spiritual distress is recognized most readily in the dying. Since death represents the final challenge to spiritual health and healing, it is no accident that the finest advances in spiritual care have come from the pioneering work of the hospice movement. Yet spiritual care cannot be seen as merely the last refuge for the hopeless case. The experience of hopelessness is a major factor in many non-terminal illnesses and disabilities, not least those mental illnesses and disabilities, such as Alzheimer's disease, which are felt to be a fate worse than death. Wherever life is seriously threatened, or terribly impaired, then spiritual needs are present, and worthy of careful recognition and response. By clarifying our understanding of spiritual distress, we reach a stronger position to help those for whom 'nothing can be done'.

From the examples above, it is clear that spiritual distress may be provoked by a number of social, economic, ethical and existential pressures. Such syndromes illustrate some of the degrading and dehumanizing factors which are common to many experiences of illness and dis-ease. Yet because these factors are ignored in the purely scientific model of disease, they may sadly go unrecognized in medical practice. It is for this reason that a deeper understanding of spirituality is an essential complement to the scientific mind.

Spirituality and doctors: a sense of vocation

'The practice of medicine is an art, not a trade; a calling, not a business; a calling in which your heart will be exercised equally with your head.' That was how Sir William Osler, one of the founding fathers of medical education, described the practice of medicine to his students at the turn of the century (Osler 1892).

Today, the sense of 'calling' or 'vocation' has become taboo. The spirituality of health care professionals is deemed to be a private matter which should not interfere with the objectivity or impartiality with which they practice their profession. The concept of 'vocation' is regarded by many young doctors as at best old-fashioned, and at worst either patronizing, naïve, hypocritical or downright exploitative. It is no longer a popular ideal.

In January 1996, the British Medical Association surveyed 800 practising doctors in the United Kingdom, and found an alarming decline in the professed sense of vocation. Whereas one in six of the doctors aged over 55 saw medicine as a vocation, the proportion for younger doctors (aged under 30) was a mere one in a hundred (BMA 1995).

Such bald statistics point to a problem without explaining the underlying shift of values. In my own research amongst Christian doctors, who were generally eager to own the concept of vocation, there was still a remarkable confusion and embarrassment about the vocational ideal in modern medical practice (Whipp 1997). For some, this was simply a matter of language. 'Vocation' was rejected as a quaint and old-fashioned term, for which a significant proportion of doctors chose to use inverted commas. For others, 'vocation' was a very slippery concept which most of those questioned found very difficult to define, and some regarded as a misleading concept wide open to abuse in situations where medical goodwill is susceptible to exploitation.

This kind of research confirms the widespread concern that the quality of vocation is no longer something that can be taken for granted in health care professionals. The spirituality of vocational choice and commitment is neither understood nor uniformly respected within the scientific world view of our secular society. This suggests that the nurturing of a contemporary spirituality of vocation should become an urgent priority.

The theology of vocation

Historically speaking, the theology of human vocation was defined most clearly at the time of the Protestant reformation. Martin Luther vigorously opposed the mediaeval notion that vocation was restricted to the religious life — as if monks and nuns had 'callings' while the rest of the world merely had 'jobs'. 'Be the monks and nuns ever so holy,' he wrote, 'they have not one whit more of a calling than the rustic in the field, or the housewife going about her household tasks in the home'.

The Puritans enlarged this secular concept of calling with their doctrine of the Primary and Secondary Call. The primary call was the essential call to each person to believe and trust in God. The secondary call embraced all that was to be undertaken in the world in response to faith, harnessing each particular gift and opportunity for the service of others and the fulfilment of God-given potential. Life and work, whether secular or religious, was to be consecrated to God in the spirit of the New Testament ethic: 'Whatever you are doing, put your whole heart into it, as if you were doing it for the Lord and not for men' (Colossians 3:23).

Such a lofty vision of vocation had far-reaching social consequences. The vigour that was let loose into society, with the blessing of reformed theology, spawned centuries of commercial and professional expansion, not least in the field of health care and development. Medical pioneers, like the Quaker Thomas Hodgkin, renowned for his study of lymph glands, or the Roman Catholic Theophile Laennec, inventor of the stethoscope, saw themselves fulfilling the work of God. Even as recently as 1833, the neurologist Charles Bell, remembered for the facial palsy which bears his name, could give the following title to his doctoral thesis: 'The hand, its mechanisms and vital endowments, as evincing the power, wisdom and goodness of God'.

Today, most doctors would be embarrassed by such an overtly theological profession of vocation. Despite the deep privilege and quiet sense of wonder which is felt by anyone engaged in human healing, today's doctors find it exceedingly difficult to voice their vocational joy and commitment in spiritual terms. The scientific mindset, with its shallow materialism and calculating utilitarianism, has squeezed out the more sensitive and spiritual intuition of a uniquely special vocation.

The ethic of vocation

Part of our problem is due to a deeply unbalanced work ethic. The Protestant Reformers, who promoted such a splendid theology of secular work, had no equivalent theology of rest. The legacy of the Protestant Work Ethic in our own time is not the glad commitment to worthwhile work which the Puritans sought to inspire, but the grinding workaholism of a society which has remembered all the material benefits of hard work and long hours, whilst forgetting the spiritual value of inner rest and peace.

As a result, our health care professions are plagued by overwork. Stress, burnout and alcohol abuse are disproportionately high, as the consuming public demands from its doctors and nurses an ever-increasing quantity of health care interventions, rather than the personal quality of a healthy and well-ordered life.

It is the 'fix-it' mentality of the scientific and technological era that has encouraged this unhealthy obsession with quantity over quality. The pinnacle of scientific efficiency in today's cost-conscious health service is the utilization of every available minute for treatment, so that no patient should be kept waiting. This greedy approach to time and technology is in stark contrast to the restful philosophy of eastern Ayurvedic physicians, who preserve two to three hours of contemplation time each day before embarking on patient care.

The support of vocation

Authentic spirituality can never be hurried. It takes time to nurture the gentleness and compassion of the healing vocation. Where science rushes for results, spirituality rests on the need for wholeness. Martha, in her busy utilitarianism, needs to learn from Mary's stillness and spiritual receptivity.

It is sad to see how doctors are sometimes their own worst enemies, in colluding with impossible workloads and innumerable commitments — all in the name of increased 'health'! They need the support of church and colleagues and friends if they are ever to make time to pause, and ponder and prayerfully rediscover their true vocation.

It is interesting to see the idea of 'reflective practice' being introduced into current management thinking. This contemplative approach to vocation is something that should be central to the spirituality of any worthwhile profession. A recent pastoral letter from Ireland offered the following helpful reflection on the theme of vocational choice and commitment:

'What can I do?'
Respect that question.
Trust that you, one man, one woman,
can do for God what otherwise would not be done.
Trust that some people will hear the gospel of Jesus,
that some who are in need will find the touch of human love,
that others will find a listening ear or a voice in their poverty,
only because you have chosen to give God
a central place in your life…
It is not just your work, your choice, your decision.
You choose because you are chosen,
you choose because in the heart of your desire to love,
you have found the heart of God searching for you.

(Irish Bishops 1989)

Spirituality and society: a culture of care

Within a national health service, the individual vocation to heal is harnessed within the framework of a vast caring institution. The spirituality of individuals is only realized within the wider context of the caring ethic of our whole society.

In Britain, this caring ethic has been profoundly influenced by Christianity. As we have seen, the organization of health care began in the monasteries. Since those first beginnings, each voluntary or state provision has reflected to some extent the Judaeo-Christian commitment to neighbourly care.

It was this commitment that inspired the Beveridge report to challenge the five giants of idleness, poverty, squalor, ignorance and disease. The National Health Service was first conceived as a Christian social institution, providing health care from the cradle to the grave, to every member of society, free at the point of need.

There is no doubt that the welfare state did much to enshrine fundamental Christian principles, embodying the Gift Relationship ('freely you have received, freely give …') in which care is offered with no regard to payment. Yet, equally, there is little doubt that the generosity of such ubiquitous caring has been abused. In retrospect, we can see that Beveridge was naïve. The insurance budget to maintain the service was grossly underestimated. Beveridge optimistically assumed that, as diseases were treated, so the demand for health care would decline. The reverse now seems to be true. With every advance in knowledge, and every new application of technology, we find that the demand for treatment, and the population in need of care, continues to increase. We have reached a point of such insatiable demand that a simplistic ideal of caring can no longer be sustained.

'Teach us to care, and not to care,' wrote T. S. Eliot in a prayer that faces the honest limits of all human caring, and refuses to divorce opportunity from cost constraints (Eliot 1963).

It is a question of stewardship. Genuine care requires both an infinite commitment to the individual, and an intricate concern for the just ordering of society. The latter is exemplified in the meticulous details of Old Testament ethics, in which the social and economic practicalities of living together as a caring community are spelled out in the context of divine covenant. The former is seen superbly in the New Testament ethic, where stories such as the Good Samaritan illustrate how compassion for one individual in need overrides every other human priority.

The challenge is to hold these opposing poles in tension, combining individual compassion with social justice in a culture of care which is able to be generous without recklessness. This is the balance that has been lost as British culture has capitulated to market forces. By 'letting the market decide', both politicians and health care professionals have abdicated their responsibility for shaping a contemporary culture of care.

To reclaim this culture in the midst of rapid change requires a renewal of public spirituality. Baroness Macfarlane takes the prophetic vision of Micah as her framework for a renewed British culture of care:

This is what Yahweh asks of you, only this,
that you act justly [an obligation to share resources equitably],
love tenderly [a call to compassion],
and walk humbly with your God [renewing spirituality at its source].

(Micah 6:8)

THE ALTERNATIVE AGENDA

The revival of spirituality might awaken some strange bedfellows, however. It is an extraordinary paradox that, at a time when the achievements of medical science are greater than they have ever been, patients should be voting against it with their feet, by turning away from scientific medicine to alternative therapies of various kinds.

Patients are looking for something more spiritual, and they will seek out any alternative from Acupuncture to Zen in their quest for holistic healing. It is no accident that in the era of maximum technological potential we are witnessing an upsurge of interest in primitive therapies which address the most basic human needs for kindness and comfort, touch and time.

This stampede towards alternative therapy represents a rejection of the impersonality of scientific medicine, which is phenomenally clever at doing things *to* people, but distressingly bad at being present *for* them. Alternative therapies offer human meaning, value and relationship, and they put the patient back in control. In many ways, they supply the missing spiritual dimension that has been driven out by the mechanistic scientific mind.

However, not every alternative is benign. Some come packaged in all kinds of bizarre theories, diets and rituals, sometimes mixed with pseudo-scientific jargon, sometimes with a smattering of the occult. Some unfairly criticize proven and effective treatments, whilst falsely promoting their own dubious claims to success. Some, worst of all, exploit the vulnerable for emotional or even financial gain.

Most complementary therapies are practised in a spirit of great compassion and sensitivity, and they have a great deal to offer in redressing the balance towards spirituality in the predominantly scientific domain of health care. There can be problems, however, due to a lack of honest criticism. The stringent evaluation of therapeutic efficacy that is mandatory for mainstream medicine can be avoided or even twisted by alternative enthusiasts in their flight from logic to magic. The result, despite all good intentions, can be seriously irrational and sadly unethical. This is the danger of a naïve search for 'spirituality' without an accompanying critical, even scientific, sense of truth.

THE APPLIANCE OF SCIENCE

The scientific mind is sincerely committed to truth. Despite the blinkers that dull the brightness of wonder and mystery, the redeeming virtue of the scientific method is its humble dependence upon proof. Personal conviction and wishful thinking carry no weight without clear and convincing *evidence* that what is being claimed is rooted in reality.

In the field of spirituality and health care, the most helpful contribution of the scientist is a humble and healthy scepticism. That is not to deny that there are mysteries that transcend rational enquiry, but to defend the truth against nonsense, mumbo-jumbo and disreputable quackery. In their common commitment to truth, spirituality and science stand side by side.

Science asks for honest answers to honest questions. How may the insights of spirituality best be applied in the care of the sick? What is the diagnostic profile of spiritual distress? And what are its most common presenting symptoms? What are the factors that undermine professional vocation, and how can they be avoided? Can we measure the outcomes of spiritual care? And how should we evaluate the benefit of training in spiritual awareness and support? In all these ways, the critical questions of the scientific mind can point the way to better practice in a faithful and honest application of spirituality to patient care.

SOME WAYS FORWARD

The characterization of spiritual dis-ease

The work presented in this book represents one important contribution to this important and neglected area of clinical competence. It is interesting that health purchasers are currently seeking criteria by which to evaluate the provision of spiritual care at every level of the service. They will need a much clearer appreciation of the scope of spiritual dis-ease and the standards of spiritual support if they are going to define best practice.

Likewise, health educators are looking for guidance on the content and approach to training in spiritual care. It is being recognized that spirituality and the spiritual dimension of health can be taught, not sheepishly, but sensitively, within an atmosphere of open-minded scientific enquiry.

In the characterization of what is meant by spiritual dis-ease, and the clarification of what is involved in spiritual care, we face a very important challenge to the combined insights of spirituality and the scientific mind.

The restoration of medical vocation

As the year 2000 approaches, the medical profession is soberly reviewing its core values for the 21st century (BMA 1994). The uncertain sense of vocation is seeking clearer articulation in this contemporary quest for spiritual and moral benchmarks. At a time of dizzying change in the social and economic context of medical practice, it is not surprising that the leaders of the profession should be re-examining their foundations.

From the debate so far, the key values that have emerged include compassion, caring, competence, and a spirit of open enquiry — a powerful blend of spirituality and the scientific mind. It is a serious debate, which has been met by more encouragement than scepticism thus far. There is a mood of seriousness, even soul-searching, in many quarters of the profession, where the loss of an intangible sense of vocation is keenly felt, particularly amongst the young.

What is lacking, however, is the sense of confidence that comes from a living spiritual tradition that is shared across society. Without spiritual renewal in this larger and more prophetic dimension, it is unlikely that BMA pronouncements will inspire much hope.

The renewal of public care

The crisis of spirituality in Britain is a crisis at the source. Our society has lost confidence in the traditional roots of spirituality that are found in the Christian and other faith traditions. The result is a loss of vocation, a weakened sense of the common good, and a growing anxiety to protect individual and sectional interests.

In the recent history of the health service, this trend can be seen in the domination of scientific economism over the broader human concerns for justice and compassion. We have lost the vision of caring stewardship which inspired the concept of the Gift Relationship in public life.

At this critical stage of fragmentation in the British culture of care, it is vital for spirituality and economic science to search for a common language in which to plead for the common good.

CONCLUSION: THE DOCTOR'S DILEMMA

George Bernard Shaw, in his famous preface to *The Doctor's Dilemma*, observed that 'doctors, if no better than other men, are certainly no worse'.

In today's society, they face enormous tensions between the claims of science, and the challenge of spirituality — for their patients, for the health service, and, not least, for themselves. In giving due respect to both, there is hope in the prayer of Sir Robert Hutchison published in the *British Medical Journal* in 1953:

From inability to leave well alone;
From too much zeal for what is new and contempt for what is old;
From putting knowledge before wisdom, science before art,
  cleverness before common sense;
From treating patients as cases; and
From making the cure of a disease more grievous than its endurance,
  Good Lord, deliver us.

REFERENCES

BMA 1994 Core values for the medical profession. British Medical Association, London
BMA 1995 BMA cohort study of 1995 medical graduates. British Medical Association, London, p 5
Eliot T S 1963 Ash Wednesday. In: Collected poems 1909–1962. Faber & Faber, London, p 105
Irish Bishops 1989 Come, follow me: Pastoral of the Irish Bishops. Quoted in: Neary D 1994 Forty masses with young people. The Columba Press, Dublin, p 123
Macfarlane J 1995 The culture of care: Christians and the changing face of public health. Lecture to the Institute of Contemporary Christianity, London
Osler W 1892 The principles and practice of medicine. Oxford University Press, Oxford, p 1
Whipp M J 1997 A healthy sense of vocation? Contact 122: 3–10

The notion of spiritual care in professional practice

Anne Johnson

INTRODUCTION

Many health service carers feel that there is an element missing in the care they deliver. Patients have become customers and staff have become human resources. The therapeutic bond that develops between patient and carer when truly holistic care is delivered has been weakened. Spiritual care is the missing element, and carers must learn how to deal with the spirituality of their patients and themselves. This chapter identifies and attempts to resolve some of the problems that this raises.

The first part of the chapter will concentrate on the existing situation with regard to the education of health care professionals in the area of spiritual care. It will look at the difficulties of defining what is meant by spiritual care and therefore designing curricula that deal with this very complicated subject. This will lead on to looking at ways in which spiritual care needs can be identified by staff and incorporated into a care plan, thus providing a much more holistic approach to care. The relationship between spiritual and physical/psychological problems will also be discussed, including the ways in which the resolution of one may well negate the other.

The chapter will end by looking at how an institution such as a large district general hospital trust can develop a training strategy for all levels and disciplines of staff that will ensure spiritual care is given equal priority when it comes to the care and treatment of its patients.

THE CURRENT SITUATION

In today's ever-changing, multicultural and rapid-turnover health service, many health care professionals already struggle to provide the holistic type of care that meets their patients' bio-psychosocial needs. Adding another dimension, spiritual care, may seem just too difficult to cope with. After all, how will staff assess their patients' spiritual needs and just where will they find the extra time and other resources that this aspect of care will require? The pre-registration training of most health care professionals will not have prepared them for this facet of care. Where spiritual care has been referred to, it will often sit alongside religious and cultural needs in a curriculum and therefore be seen as being dealt with by an appropriate religious leader to whom patients are often referred. A hospital chaplain will often 'teach' this part of a curriculum, and in the minds of the students this will define spirituality as religion. This is the crux of the problem when it comes to educating staff in all aspects of spiritual care: the definition of what it really means. The fact that there are no physical tests or easy ways of finding out what a patient's spiritual needs are makes it all the more difficult to embed it into a philosophy of care and educational programmes that equip people to give that care.

If spiritual care is not dealt with adequately in pre-registration programmes, can one then assume that post-registration training programmes will cover the subject? I suspect not. They will deal with the many of the skills required to make a spiritual needs assessment, such as communication and interpersonal skills, counselling and observation skills, but they are unlikely to make the connection specifically with spiritual care, and therefore will not raise the awareness of practitioners and help them to understand that spiritual care is just as important as physical care or dealing with psychological problems. The exception to this is possibly in the field of palliative care education, where a more holistic approach to care may be taken.

Nurses are taught about a number of models of care that act as a framework on which to assess patients' care needs. One of the most commonly used models, *The Elements of Nursing* (Roper, Logan & Tierney 1996), does not identify spiritual needs as an entity in their own right. The model looks at the Activities of Living in a fairly task-oriented way. It briefly touches on the influence of religion and refers to ethnic and cultural differences that may affect the way patients are nursed. The model describes how religious beliefs may affect a patient's attitude towards health, but it goes no further in looking at other spiritual influences that should be taken into account when caring for patients.

UNDERSTANDING WHAT IS MEANT BY SPIRITUAL CARE

So how do we deal with spiritual needs in a health care setting? First of all we have to define what we mean by spiritual. We all have spiritual needs even though we may not recognize them as such. Many individuals, practitioners and patients will feel that because they do not see themselves as a religious person they do not have spiritual needs. Religious and cultural beliefs and practices are an important part of the spiritual dimension, but there are other aspects that should not be forgotten. Many patients will invest time and energy into other areas that give their life purpose and meaning. When they become ill these areas are affected too, and carers must learn to recognize and deal with the difficulties that this will bring. Carers should explore their own spirituality and develop an awareness of their needs although they are often reluctant to do this. Wilfred McSherry (1996) recognizes that spiritual awareness may imply religiosity or piety rather than the ability to explore one's attitudes and feelings. He goes on to say that for nurses to understand, explore and offer spiritual support to their patients, they must gain this insight into the spiritual dimension of care.

When trying to help people to understand this, we may ask them what is important in their lives, what gives them purpose or meaning, or what gives them the strength to carry on? The answers we get back will range from religion to a favourite football team, from a career to a well-tended garden, from a beloved pet to a beloved partner. All of these answers show the diversity of the spiritual dimension and the difficulties inherent in trying to deal with spiritual issues as a routine part of care.

Most of us are motivated by the need to feel fulfilled; we want more than just a safe existence, we want to develop to our fullest potential. Maslow's hierarchy of needs (Maslow 1954) reflects this in what he calls self-actualization. However, when we are ill, whatever form that illness takes, our most pressing needs are often physical or possibly psychological. This is the case with our patients. Their need to understand the illness and treatment will probably be more powerful initially than any other need. Their anxiety or fear may well be the overriding emotion, and thoughts of spiritual needs will fade into the background as they cope with the physical threat that their illness may pose to them.

Health care professionals will identify with their patients' needs and make every effort to assess, diagnose and treat the physical and psychological problems whilst not necessarily recognizing that the spiritual needs even exist. These needs therefore will remain unmet for the duration of the patient's illness.

Probably the best way of providing that truly holistic approach to care is to help all carers, whatever their discipline or level, to recognize the value of dealing with the spiritual dimension of care. The fact that we all have spiritual needs but don't necessarily express them can make this more difficult to handle. Carers must recognize the difficulties they have when their own spiritual needs are not met. How do they cope even though they may be physically fit, have no particular worries or problems, yet for some reason still feel unhappy? What 'snaps them out of it'? What makes it possible for them to carry on, gives them a sense of purpose and meaning, fills their life with hope? Once the carers can understand this of themselves they can use this knowledge when caring for their patients and try to take account of spiritual care needs as a part of the caring process.

THE PROCESS OF CARING FOR SPIRITUAL NEEDS

The process of care in the spiritual dimension is no different from that in any other. It requires a comprehensive assessment of any problems or needs and a detailed care plan to resolve the problems.

The nursing process comprises four simple steps:

- assessment
- planning
- implementation
- evaluation.

These four steps can be used when preparing a plan of care for a patient's spiritual needs. This plan should be a part of the overall care plan for the patient and not seen as separate, for in reality spiritual needs are usually inextricably linked with physical and psychological needs.

Assessment

This is the first and possibly the most difficult step of the process, and it has been examined elsewhere in this book (Ch. 8). Most professional carers use a variety of assessment tools or frameworks on which to base a physical or psychological assessment. These are very few and far between in the spiritual field. Where they do exist, and are used, there is always the danger of assuming that if we have asked the right questions, or have followed a particular framework rigidly, then we will have done a good assessment. One example of an assessment tool can be found in the document *A Framework for Spiritual Faith and Related Pastoral Care* (Institute of Nursing, University of Leeds

1995). Here it is suggested that in an interview-type situation there are four distinct areas that should be addressed: worship, religious health care issues, death, and everyday customs. It also says that although the issue of death is a spiritual one, it should be dealt with separately from the other so as not to cause distress to a patient. Whilst this assessment tool is fine as far as it goes, a spiritual needs assessment will usually be more complex. The experience and professional judgement of carers will come into play. A comprehensive assessment is not something that can be completed in a one-off situation when the initial admissions process is taking place.

The patient and carer have to build up a relationship of mutual trust and respect before a patient will feel able to divulge his or her more 'personal' issues to the carer. Because of the diversity of the human condition, the building of this relationship may take a long time, or it may be very rapid depending on the patient's situation. Whatever that situation, the carer has to use all of his or her skills to make a comprehensive assessment of the patient's needs. Assessment skills include listening, observing, communication and interpersonal skills.

Listening

The carer has to listen not only to what the patient says but also to how he says it. The tone of voice, the speed at which it is said and what is happening when it is being said are all important. The carer must also be aware of how the patient is communicating with her family, and might talk to relatives and friends in order to acquire a fuller picture of the patient. It will help the carer to judge whether or not the patient is troubled by something.

Observing

Non-verbal cues may give us the key to the patient's spiritual wellbeing. Sometimes what is said is belied by a gesture or a look. Observation of patients when they are alone or with their families, and when they are not being formally assessed, may also give us information that we may not otherwise obtain. The patient's response to information and treatment should also be observed carefully. For example, on hearing bad news about his prognosis or after undergoing a particularly difficult treatment, a patient may well show some indication of a spiritual need that has not previously been identified. This will sometimes manifest itself as something that would previously have been out of character. It is perhaps not so surprising that many patients find some comfort in some religious format when their physical being is threatened. In today's multicultural, multiethnic society, this may take many forms, and carers have to be aware of the different requirements of all of their patients.

Communication and interpersonal skills

Good skills in these areas are essential. A carer must be sure that she is communicating well with her patients so that a relationship of trust can be developed as soon as possible. A patient often 'hands over' her welfare to the caring team on admission to hospital and expects to be able to rely on them, to be well cared for and informed about her condition. Helping patients to understand their own situation and therefore help in the assessment process can only be done by good communication.

Assessment, then, is very difficult. It will often take precious time that, in a health service where time is a particularly scarce resource, may well be seen by some carers as a luxury that they can't afford. However, carers should understand that assessing for spiritual needs is not done in isolation. It is probably best done when undertaking other 'tasks' or it may simply be the result of passing the time of day with a patient or relative. It is the role of everyone in the care team to pick up the cues, comments and direct requests and pass on information to their colleagues so that a comprehensive assessment can take place.

It is worth remembering that care is only as good as the care plan and that the care plan is only as good as the assessment of needs.

Planning

Planning care should come as second nature once the need for care has been established and stated in a care plan. If only the process were so simple! A broken leg, the need for information, or the delivery of a drug are easily expressed in a written care plan. To some degree they are standardized and can be undertaken by specific members of the caring team. The spiritual care plan, however, will be much more difficult to articulate. To start with, the expression of the problem or need may not be easy, particularly if it is related to a feeling or emotion displayed by the patient. For example, the need to feel like an individual rather than a hospital number with a medical condition is something we should all understand, but how many of us relate this to specific patient needs? The care required may be equally difficult to put into words in a written care plan.

Spiritual problems or needs may often be identified on care plans as part of so-called psychological problems. For example, a patient may be assessed as being anxious about going to theatre, but what is behind that anxiety? The real problem may be that the patient is worried about being unable to do some of the things that made his life worth living prior to the operation, rather than worried about the pain or the anaesthetic — which is how he may have expressed his anxiety. Therefore finding the right words to state the problem or need should be discussed with the patient.

Sometimes spiritual care planning is about good communication between members of the care team. Passing on information and the patients' thoughts and feelings within the boundaries of confidentiality is very important and can't always be done in writing. The value of case conferences, oral reports and discussion is evident in many cases. The professional carers, the patient and their family/friends should have opportunities to discuss any spiritual problems or needs and be able to look for ways to resolve problems together. Professional carers often see themselves as experts in planning, but in the case of spiritual care it may often be someone who knows the patient well, an informal carer or family member, who is the best person to view the situation and with help suggest a plan of care that will be acceptable to the patient.

Implementation

Bringing to fruition a plan of care is a skilled task. Needs and care must be prioritized so that the right care is given at the right time. Care often becomes task oriented and compartmentalized so that there is a start and end point. The delivery of spiritual care is often a much more ongoing process. It builds up over a period of time as the patient and carers get to know one another. In a formal care setting, such as a hospital ward or department, patients are often cared for by an extensive team of professionals with whom any one interaction may take only a few minutes. Even within nursing where the patient has a so-called 'named nurse' the constancy of the relationship between patient and nurse cannot be guaranteed and care can become fragmented.

This will lead to the patient's feeling unsatisfied and even apprehensive without being able to state why. For this reason spiritual care is implemented alongside physical care; it becomes a natural part of the caring process and is the responsibility of all members of the caring team.

Of course there may well be times when resolving a patient's spiritual care needs will be more important than resolving physical ones. This is probably where the professional judgement of the carer comes to the fore and there is a realization that dealing with a spiritual problem may well help to resolve a physical or psychological problem. This has been supported by research. For example, in the field of pain control, Hayward (1975) identified the patient's need for information and to understand their pain. Where the patient is informed and aware of what to expect and understands how the pain will be overcome, it is often the case that the pain can be controlled much better by the patient, and the need for drug therapy may be reduced. The patient needs to have some control over the process in order to be as self-managing as possible. This is also be the case with spiritual needs. In the example highlighted in the Planning subsection, above, where a patient is worried about being able to return to a normal life after an operation, this patient's problem can be dealt with preoperatively. The patient may for example, feel that his life would not be worth living if he couldn't continue with his hobby of playing golf. Looking at the physical constraints that the operation may put on the patient, and helping the patient to deal with them before they become a problem, will probably make the patient's physical recovery much quicker.

Sometimes when dealing with spiritual problems the professional carers have to defer to the patient's greater knowledge on how to deal with a problem once it has been identified. Hierarchies that often develop in the formal caring teams may be broken down when fulfilling spiritual needs. It may not be the team leader or most highly qualified member of staff that is best placed to deliver spiritual care. It is clear that in these days of finite resources and increasing patient activity a large proportion of a patient's 'hands-on' care may be given by support staff rather than professionally qualified staff. They will often spend more time with the patient and their significant others. It is particularly important then that any team leader recognizes this and helps to facilitate it. The importance of all members of the team must be recognized in order to ensure that all aspects of care are delivered to the highest standard.

Evaluation

To close the circle of the caring process the care given must be evaluated, the care plan reviewed and changed if required. It is hard to evaluate the effectiveness of spiritual care. There are probably only a small number of standards that can be audited, and therefore evaluation is often an imprecise process. Where there are standards, for example in the first national Charter Standard of the Patient's Charter (Department of Health 1991), they can be formally audited. Some health care providers will also refer to the spiritual dimension in their general philosophy of care. However, when it comes to evaluating an individual patient's care, the carer can take his cues from the patient. The effects of spiritual care will probably be expressed by the patient as a feeling of wellbeing, being in control or simply not feeling anxious about their care — the feeling of 'getting back to normal'. This feeling can prevail even though the patient's physical progress may not be so good and in some cases where the prognosis is very bad. The difficulty in evaluating spiritual care is that it is often not a case of cause and effect. It can't be compared to having a headache, taking a pill and waiting for the headache to go away. It is very much more complex than that, it is usually very subjective on both the patient's and the carer's part and is often linked with other aspects of physical care that can't be teased apart. This makes it much more difficult to decide whether or not one has been successful. When trying to evaluate spiritual care the carer should go back to the beginning and reassess the patient's spiritual needs and compare this assessment with the initial one. Discussion with the patient is the most obvious way of doing this, together with observation of the patient. Does the patient react to the environment in the same way as when she was admitted? Is she more able to ask questions and express her problems? Can she communicate more readily? Does she seem more at ease? These are the sorts of questions that should be asked.

PUTTING SPIRITUAL CARE ON THE AGENDA

In order to develop any sort of educational strategy that deals with spiritual care in a large district general hospital-type setting, one first needs to get spiritual care on the agenda of both the senior managers at board level and the purchasers at district health authority level. The National Association of Health Authorities and Trusts, in its document *Spiritual Care in the NHS*

— *a Guide for Purchasers and Providers* (National Association of Health Authorities and Trusts 1996) have attempted to do this. The document explores action that should be undertaken by both providers and purchasers of health care. Health care provision is currently based on business principles as much as on caring principles. It is provided via a series of contracts between health authorities or general practitioners and trusts. Within these contracts, health care providers have to meet quality specifications at both local and national level. Spiritual care is very much a quality issue that is very difficult to measure, but one is unlikely to find reference to it within the contracts as a quality indicator. The Patient's Charter refers to privacy, dignity and religious and cultural beliefs; it states:

The Charter Standard is that all health services should make provision so that proper personal consideration is shown to you, for example by ensuring that your privacy, dignity and religious and cultural beliefs are respected. Practical arrangements should include meals to suit all your dietary requirements and private rooms for confidential discussions with relatives. (Department of Health 1991)

This in itself does not cover spiritual care in its entirety, but it is a starting point from which some purchasers could begin to develop measurable quality outcome indicators. The purchaser should also be checking on such areas as the education of staff and the place that spiritual care has in the mission statement of the health care provider. Senior managers and board members have a responsibility to ensure that spiritual issues are recognized as an important part of the institution's quality programme. They should become part of the trust's core objectives. An education strategy should be developed and endorsed by the board to ensure that spiritual care is seen as high on the agenda. Clinicians have a responsibility to raise the issue at any venue where the people with these responsibilities may listen.

DEVELOPING AN EDUCATION STRATEGY

Developing a strategy to introduce the concept of spiritual care will be a complex and time-consuming process with many stages (see Fig. 11.1) It is about changing the culture of an organization and the individuals that work within it. The process begins by finding some champions, people who have an interest in the subject and, one hopes, a better degree of understanding. This group can be formed into a steering group, preferably chaired by a board member or senior manager within the establishment. The

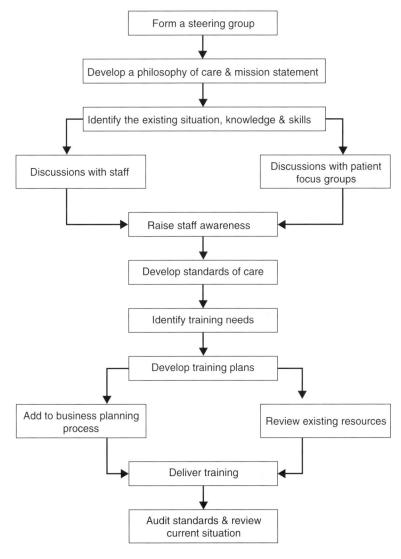

Figure 11.1   Development of a strategy to introduce the concept of spiritual care.

group should be multidisciplinary and comprise both junior and senior members of staff. If patients can be represented on the group, it will add greatly to the credibility of its work. The steering group should begin by formulating a philosophy of care and a mission statement for the trust that will provide a focus for its work.

Identifying the current situation within the trust is the next piece of work that must be undertaken. This is an information-gathering exercise where representative groups of staff will be interviewed and patient focus groups formed to encourage discussions where opinions and good ideas can be canvassed. The result of the information gathering will be a benchmark that will help to evaluate any education strategy that is put into place.

Once a benchmark has been established, the steering group must begin to raise the awareness and profile of spiritual issues among its staff. The philosophy and mission statement should be widely publicized. Through a series of seminars or discussion groups and also by adding the issue to the agendas of existing groups, information can be made available to carers. Educating staff in providing spiritual care is very much like educating staff in customer care or health and safety issues. It is everybody's business, and all staff have a responsibility with regard to it. If spiritual care is to become part of the core purpose of the organization then it should be seen to be as important as these other areas. Including it in the philosophy and mission statement will begin the long process of changing the culture of the organization and its staff.

An education programme should be aimed at different levels and different staff groups. The things to be taken into account when doing this will be existing skills, previous training and possibly how much direct patient contact time each group has.

Staff could be divided into three main groups:

- administration and clerical
- clinical support
- 'hands-on' clinical.

Administration and clerical would comprise telephonists, secretarial and other staff whose interaction with patients may well be very fleeting, on a fairly superficial level, and who are therefore unlikely to develop a specific relationship with the patient. Clinical support staff may spend either longer periods of time with the patients or have a series of short encounters with them that enable them to build up some sort of relationship. This group would include ward receptionists, physiotherapists and other technical staff. The third group would be those staff working in ward teams and who provide the majority of hands-on patient care. This is probably the largest category and would comprise nursing and medical staff at different levels.

Once these groups have been agreed, their differing training needs can be identified, deciding which groups of staff need what skills and at what level. For example, good communication is at the heart of good care. All staff can be helped to improve their communication skills, from senior managers to ancillary/support staff, whereas counselling skills are very specialized and counselling is probably best left to a few experts. Some education will be undertaken at local level and may well consist of a short 1 or 2 day course, or it may be more appropriate to cover an issue of training by using longer and academically accredited programmes.

RESOURCES FOR EDUCATION

Once an education strategy has been developed, it must be realistically costed. Education is expensive both in time and money, and there are often hidden costs that are not apparent initially. The cost of tutor time and time out for staff must be estimated, together with any specific course fees. Whether or not staff have to be replaced in clinical areas is also something that must be considered. Funds for training can be accessed from organizations outside of the trust. For example, at a vocational level, training will often be funded either in part or totally by local Chambers of Commerce, Training and Enterprise. The newly constituted Health Service Regional Education Consortia will also have a role to play in obtaining funding. One of their main functions is to contract with the education providers on behalf of health care providers for post-basic education programmes to fulfil their needs. The consortia also hold regional budgets that fund the contracts. They will become invaluable not only for providing funds but also in influencing education providers in the type of programmes that they provide.

As most organizations will have limited resources, it may also be wise to prioritize training and development. Decide which group of staff is most in need, and have the costs identified as part of the business planning processes which is essential to the success of an education strategy. The development and delivery of education programmes will probably be spread over a long period of time as time is also a scarce resource. However, once the education strategy becomes embedded in the organization, the final stage of the process can begin. The standards that have been developed will be audited and the benchmark revisited so that the current situation at that time can be reviewed. The circle of education and audit will become a dynamic, continuous process that will enable the trust to maintain and enhance its standards of patient care.

STAFF SUPPORT

Caring for patients can be very stressful both physically and mentally. Expanding care to meet patients' spiritual needs may well increase that stress and can be a very emotional process for the carer. It is very easy for staff to take on the problems of their patients when they are providing support day after day, often not only for the patient but also for the family and friends as well. This can lead to excessive amounts of stress and so-called burnout. Before staff get to this point, their work (and personal life) will be affected in various ways that reduce their effectiveness. These could include:

- difficulty in concentrating
- bad timekeeping
- forgetfulness
- poor decision making
- high sickness levels
- depressed performance generally.

Stress has become an everyday part of the working life of most people. It is in the interests of any employer to help its staff manage that stress. In many respects, informal support systems can be very effective. Time out for staff in a social setting is often a good way to relieve stress. Talking over problems and discussing feelings is sometimes best done with staff who experience those same problems and feelings and can empathize. However, these types of informal system may also bring their own problems with them. Staff sometimes feel that admitting to problems is a sign of weakness, failure to cope and shows an inability to do the job well. For an organization to help its staff deal with this, it must develop a culture whereby staff feel able to disclose their difficulties and know that there will be a number of non-judgemental support systems available to them.

Educating staff to understand spiritual issues and deal with the spiritual care needs of their patients will in itself help to reduce the stress. Carers will feel less inadequate and therefore more able to provide the desired standard of care.

Access to a confidential telephone helpline may assist staff to unburden themselves of some of the everyday pressures that they constantly encounter. Sometimes a situation requires a face-to-face discussion with a trusted mentor. Clinical supervision, although the title may not suggest it, can be a very supportive relationship. It provides a safe and confidential arena in which the supervisee can reflect on their practice and discuss potential solutions. It can also be an educative process where an experienced supervisor can give the supervisee the benefit of that experience. By sharing problems and solutions, the subject of spiritual care gradually becomes less difficult to deal with. Phil Barker (1996) makes the point that if nurses fail to recognize their own vulnerability, it may only serve to make that vulnerability worse and it might further undermine their mental wellbeing and reduce the value of the therapeutic relationship between patient and carer.

If stress has not been dealt with either informally or through a clinical supervision relationship, it will begin to affect not only the person's work ability but also their physical health. At this point the person must be referred to a trained counsellor. This will probably be done through the organization's occupational health department.

Lastly, carers must learn to look after their own colleagues. The signs of excessive stress have already been identified in the chapter. How many of us acknowledge them when we come across them in our fellow workers and try to help? Do we sometimes simply complain when one member of the team does not appear to be pulling their weight? Perhaps we should all be better at empathizing with our colleagues. After all it would be easy for anyone to find themselves in exactly the same place at some time or other.

CONCLUSION

In conclusion it would seem, then, that spiritual needs are often a misunderstood and therefore neglected facet of care. Both patients and staff have difficulty in understanding the concept, and currently there is little research or education that explores the area in any depth. One thing is certain: if there is to be any improvement in the situation, basic training for all groups of staff, to enable them to understand the concept, is essential. The connections between spiritual, physical, psychological and social care must be clarified and a truly holistic approach to care advocated by all health care professionals. The purchasers of health care and the strategic planners of health care provision need to have a clearer understanding of the issue and include this as an indicator in their quality specifications.

Finally, health care organizations must promote a culture in which staff feel supported and able to explore their own spirituality in order to help them understand their patients' problems. It is only by doing this that the organization can then begin to provide a high standard of truly holistic care.

REFERENCES

Barker P 1996 Working with mental distress. Nursing Times 92(2): 25–27
Department of Health 1991 The Patient's Charter. Department of Health, London
Hayward J 1975 Information: a prescription against pain. Royal College of Nursing, London
Institute of Nursing, University of Leeds, National Health Service Executive Northern Yorkshire 1995 A framework for spiritual faith and related pastoral care. Barkers, Manchester
Maslow A H 1954 Motivation of personality. Harper & Row, New York
McSherry W 1996 Raising the spirits. Nursing Times 97(3): 48–49
National Association of Health Authorities and Trusts 1996 Spiritual care in the NHS: a guide for purchasers and providers. National Association of Health Authorities and Trusts, Birmingham
Roper N, Logan W, Tierney A 1996 The elements of nursing, 4th edn. Churchill Livingstone, Edinburgh

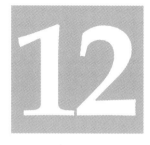

Spirituality and hospice care

Neil Small

INTRODUCTION

The history of care for the sick and dying shows a long tradition of contributions both from religious orders and from those individuals who seek to manifest their religious faith via such work. These contributions had often been closely in harmony with prevalent social beliefs but, in modern times, can appear at odds with secular, rational and scientific approaches to life and death. While there are examples of the continuation of care by religious orders, a more prevalent response has been to locate religious contributions in the person of the clergy, often acting as members of a multidisciplinary care team.

There has also been sustained and widespread development of an approach that seeks to separate the religious from the spiritual, or at least to deny that these terms ought to be considered as synonymous. In this approach the spiritual is identified with a search for meaning (Walter 1997). As such, the dimension of the spiritual is retained as a central component of care. But it is a dimension that essentially depicts a journey rather than a destination. It is the search rather than any belief that is given priority. In so doing the possibility is evoked of many different approaches to the spiritual being encouraged. These approaches may incorporate the transcendent and the existential, but they might also be collapsed into the psychological or even a rag bag of the vaguely personal. Consider a recent publication from Britain's National Association of Health Authorities and Trusts:

the acknowledgement of a person's language, culture, dietary needs, customs, anxiety and fear — or even their sense of isolation in unfamiliar surroundings — is an important component of spiritual care. (NAHAT 1997)

Within hospice care it has always been clear that spiritual care is 'not an optional extra' (Saunders 1965). Through the thirty years of the modern hospice movement a sense of the importance of the spiritual has been retained. Research published in 1995 compared hospice nurses and oncology nurses and demonstrated that the former group engage in spiritual care activities more often and felt more comfortable in so doing. They also indicate more satisfaction with the training and support they receive from employers in that provision of spiritual care (Johnston-Taylor, Amenta & Highfield 1995). Also evident in the nursing and palliative care press is a considerable interest in spiritual care, often drawing on hospice practice as a source of example. While it may be the case that general trends in the development of medicine, nursing and care more generally have impacted upon hospice structure and practice, it is also the case that a concern with the holistic and with the spiritual has moved out from hospice to wider areas of practice.

In this chapter I will examine the changing hospice world and its relationship with social change. I will also scrutinize the varied understandings of the spiritual and will critique the separation of the spiritual and the religious.

IS THERE A TRADITION OF SPIRITUAL CARE?

At first sight it appears very clear that in hospice care there is a well-established tradition of spiritual care. The first, 4th century, hospices established by Fabiola for pilgrims (drawing on the word 'hospes', originally meaning host but gradually changing to refer to strangers or guests) were clearly based on biblical texts and staffed by members of religious orders. These orders included the Knights Hospitaller of the Order of St John of Jerusalem who, in the 11th century, addressed their patients as 'Our Lords the Sick' (Lamerton 1980, p. 16).

There was, throughout the Christian world, a continuing centrality of Christian charitable institutions carrying the burden of the sick and the poor.

The Mediaeval hospices — whether the great fortress hospital of Rhodes, the elegant hospice of Beaune, or the myriad of small hospices associated with monasteries all over Europe — were dedicated to the care of the sick and the dying, and the Christian burial of the dead. Whether the traveller was a knight on the journey to Jerusalem, or a poor beggar on the journey of life, the ancient hospice was a way station, a resting place, a place of care and concern for both the body and the spirit. (Ley 1992, p. 208)

In the 19th century there were a number of small but important initiatives for the history of hospice care. In 1836 Pastor Fliedner founded the first Protestant order of deaconesses at Kaiserswerth, which carried out all the works of mercy, including caring for the dying. In 1842 Mme Jeanne Garnier, a Roman Catholic widow, founded her 'Calvaries' or Hospices for the dying in France. The subsequent establishment of Calvary Hospital, New York, owed much to the inspiration of this work.

Inspired by the vision of Mother Mary Aikenhead, the Irish Sisters of Charity opened a hospice for the dying near Dublin in 1879. The Sisters had reported awful problems for families trying to cope with the care of their dying in conditions of poverty, overcrowding and ignorance. A special kind of nursing home was needed that was quieter and smaller than an acute hospital but which had the same facilities for bedside nursing.

Since the Sisters considered death to be the beginning of a journey, a thoroughfare and not a terminus, the old name of the resting places on the pilgrimage to the Holy Land seemed the most appropriate. (Lamerton 1980, p. 17)

The Irish Sisters of Charity opened other hospices, including St Joseph's in East London. St Luke's House for the Dying Poor opened in 1893, started by Dr Howard Barrett in conjunction with the Methodist West London Mission. Other, in the main isolated, initiatives began in the 19th century. All were Christian, with the exception of the City Of Hope in California, opened by Jewish emigrés.

Other US initiatives included that begun by Rose Hawthorne, who watched her friend the poet Emma Lazarus die of cancer and wondered how the poor fared when similarly afflicted. *Rose founded an order of Dominican nuns who devoted themselves to terminal care. Their first hospice opened in New York City in 1899. The order, the 'Servants of Relief for incurable cancer', then opened six more homes in the USA.

In the period following the Second World War in the USA a group of New York social workers started 'Cancer Care Inc' to try and give support to people dying at home. In the UK the Marie Curie Foundation was set up with the aim of fighting the consequences of malignant disease. Also, through the 1950s and 1960s, culminating with the opening of St Christopher's Hospice in Sydenham, south east London in 1967, Dame Cicely Saunders

---

*One of Emma Lazarus's poems was inscribed at the foot of the Statue of Liberty. The poem, which includes those famous lines about tired, poor, huddled masses, finishes:

Send these, the homeless, tempest-tost to me,
I lift my lamp beside the golden door.

These are lines that, inadvertently, have a number of images resonant of the emerging hospice movement, the home for those on journeys, the golden door with its evocation of heaven and the motif of the lamp so resonant for nursing.

was reviewing and ultimately building on the tradition and practice of care from St Joseph's and elsewhere in her evolving vision of a modern hospice. That tradition included the spiritual, incorporated now into a concept of total care — physical, emotional, social and spiritual — responding to total pain.

St Christopher's is a community inspired and informed by Christianity. Cicely Saunders espoused a Christianity very much in keeping with that of earlier hospices. It is, she says, 'honour and not pity that we owe' our patients. 'Suffering was — and is — the place where Christ is glorified' and these patients 'respond much more to our thoughts about them than our words to them' (Saunders 1987: 4; first published in 1965).

In the *Aims and Basis* document, developed before the Hospice opened, it is clearly stated that

St Christopher's Hospice is based on the full Christian faith in God, through Christ. It's aim is to express the love of God to all who come, in every possible way; in skilled nursing and medical care, in the use of every scientific means of relieving suffering and distress ... the staff should form a community, united by a strong sense of vocation with a great diversity of outlook in a spirit of freedom. They all desire to make St Christopher's a home to all who come.

As for patients:

they too are free, and will receive spiritual help when and if they want it, from anyone they may choose ... to be of any real use [St Christopher's] must give the patients — whether they have faith or not — a sense of security: through faith in God, through Christ's victory over pain and death, through mutual fellowship, and the spirit of prayer, radiating out from the Chapel into every part of the corporate life. (St Christopher's Hospice 1988)

The subsequent development of hospices in the UK has been far ranging and speedy. Their nomenclature — St Luke's, St Anne's, St Barnabas' and so on — the architecture, even the letter headings, of hospices are a continual reminder of their Christian origins and continuing allegiance (Froggatt and Walter 1995). But the influence of Christianity on the development of hospice care in the era following the Second World War has been only one of many influences.

THE CHANGING CONTEXT OF HOSPICE CARE

A number of social changes have impacted upon the structure, practice and philosophy of hospice care and on the society in which hospice care has developed. These include the following.

Changes in social welfare provision

The development of the British Welfare State, in particular the National Health Service after 1948, displaced the historical centrality of religious, municipal, charitable and voluntary sector organizations in the provision of social care outside the home. It promoted the idea of collective altruism in addition to a system that was essentially an insurance-based approach — that is, one pays when able in order to benefit when not. The altruism was concerned with the idea that one had a responsibility to aid strangers, just as one could have an expectation that strangers would come to your aid.

For some people the welfare state became a sort of secular church. It both, paradoxically perhaps, absolved one from a sense of individual charitable obligation (although as hospices demonstrate, it did not end charitable giving) and at the same time gave one a sense of contributing to mutual aid (see Titmuss 1970). Much of the expansion of hospice care, and certainly specialist palliative care, has occurred under the aegis of the welfare state. Although this expansion can develop in such a way as to incorporate the spiritual antecedents and tradition of hospices it does not depend on such underpinnings.

The welfare state has undergone a paradigm shift since 1989, when the White Paper, *Working for Patients*, was published. The original balance between collective altruism and an insurance-based understanding of self-interest has been challenged by a reassertion of the primacy of the individual. In part this has been achieved via an ideological attack on the idea of society, which Prime Minister Thatcher famously announced 'did not exist'. In part it has been achieved by a series of financial changes to encourage people to plan for their own health, social care and educational provision and to encourage private provision of care. It has also been achieved by the division of welfare agencies into purchasers and providers and the infusion of a language of audit, quality, cost effectiveness, customers and so on. Overall the changes are often described via the shorthand of 'the market'.

These changes have set the scene such that a new cohort of hospice administrators can speak, without apparent discomfort, about 'the hospice business.'[†]

[†] An article in the *Health Service Journal* (Dix 1996) was titled 'Is God good value?'. It begins with the observation that the number of hospital chaplains has increased significantly since the introduction of market forces to the NHS. Many chaplains have been given budgets and asked to produce business plans.

Professionalization and specialization

The development of professionalization and specialization in care has been apparent in many areas of health and social care and is certainly evident in palliative care. The English National Board for Nursing awards two 'higher' qualifications for nurses. In 1987 palliative medicine was established as a specialty by the Royal College of Physicians. There are specialist journals, conferences and professorships of palliative medicine. These developments have been prompted by, and in turn have promoted, an increasing repertoire of technical interventions in palliative care.

As more of the difficult symptoms and syndromes of the terminal stages of life become potentially palliatable, will we see more examples of invasive and technological therapies being assimilated into previously low-tech hospice care? If so, does that process represent intrusive medicalisation, or the rational application of a better understood and safer therapy to a wider pool of patients who may benefit? (Ahmedzai 1993, p. 141)

The argument that it is medicalization, and as such represents a considerable threat to the original aims of the hospice movement, is well made by Biswas (1993). She argues that changes are occurring in the nature of staff commitment to hospices, in the focus on the holistic and in the overall stance taken to death and dying. More and more hospices have full-time medical directors; the doctor is no longer one of a team of equals. That doctor is, in effect, on a career grade in a specialty like any other. Along with the dominance of doctors comes a renewed focus on the medical approach, which is essentially directed at biological explanations, at pathology and at seeing parts rather than wholes as the focus for concern. Biswas quotes Penson and Fisher talking about terminal care, to help illustrate her point; they say that, 'important and demanding though it is, [terminal care] is usually the least difficult part of total care'. She asks:

least difficult for whom? I presume 'least difficult' for the doctor, certainly not for the patient, relatives, nurses, counsellors or chaplain. (Biswas 1993, p. 135)

Where there is a full-time medical director the hospice is more likely to make use of invasive procedures and patients are more likely to be referred for palliative surgery and organ donation. Such units are also more likely to be described in technical terms, a 'pain relief centre', a 'specialist medical/nursing unit', than non-technical, 'a peaceful haven', 'just like a family' (Johnson et al 1990).

Establishment and growth of the hospice movement

> Early on it was clear who the villains and the heroes were, where the challenges lay, what were the pitfalls to be avoided. There was the good work and it was easy to devote one's life. ... I think now we have passed that stage and ahead may lie many diverse paths, many confusions of a subtler nature. (Torrens 1981, p. 194)

James and Field, in a much cited article, have argued that there has been a routinization of charisma (James & Field 1992), and James (1994) has written of the maturing of the hospice movement from vision to system. There is a recognition, in these contributions to understanding the origins and then development of the modern hospice movement, that an initial reformist intent to change terminal care has been transformed, through both diversification and legitimation, into a mainstream activity. In effect this is part of the success of the hospice movement. But the question being raised is how far in achieving this success have some of the initial aims been left behind?

Bradshaw's contributions are significant here as she raises the spectre of the attenuation of the original ethical ideal that informed hospice and explores the impact of this on, particularly, the spiritual component of care (Bradshaw 1996). She quotes Weber speaking of shifts from charisma to routinization and bureaucratization:

> Specialists without spirit, sensualists without heart; this nullity imagines that it has attained a level of civilisation never before achieved. (Weber 1976, p. 182)

One can argue that the particular pattern of development of specialist palliative medicine is not automatically or unequivocally welcome in the evolution of hospices, because it may lead to an emphasis on a reductionist concern with technique or with one area of care as opposed to holistic care. It can change the orientation of those working in hospices from its being a mission to being a job and it can impact upon the place of spirituality. This is not to say that technical advance has not been welcome in modern hospices. Indeed the very identification of the post-1967 hospices as 'modern' is predicated on their engagement with research, innovation and teaching, for example in investigating and relieving symptoms; the use of opioids for terminal pain is one such crucial area (Saunders 1996).

Secularization

There is a prevailing assumption that we live in times that are increasingly becoming secularized. In looking at the specific development of hospices, this is a hard assumption to accept uncritically. First we must realize that, historically, the development of modern hospices is a recent phenomenon. Hospices developed in the late 1960s and 1970s, with rapid growth in numbers occurring in the 1980s. While it is the case that St Christopher's, and subsequent 'modern' hospices, were set up outside the established service run by religious orders, the initial St Christopher's approach was vocational and spiritual.

Second, we might characterize the 1980s not as a time of continuing secularization but rather as a period of reassertion by religious groups. We have seen the 'born-again' phenomena, we have seen the more visible and more wide ranging exercise of Islam in the West and, most notably in the USA, a vigorous incursion into politics by religious groups. This is in addition to what appears to be a continuing strong residual allegiance to the religious; more than 80% of the US population claims to be religious, and in the UK a 1990 MORI survey suggests that 88% of the UK population profess themselves Christian (discussed in Mitchell 1994). Grace Davie argued that the majority of British 'believe without belonging' to a Christian church (Davie 1994).

The development of other discourses on death

A number of alternative ways of understanding the end of life and responses to it exist alongside a spiritual one. Since the 1950s the study of death and dying, thanatology, has developed (see Feifal 1959). In part this built on psychology and psychoanalysis but also on the existential philosophies. Freud on the death instinct, death in society and on mourning and melancholy had been influential not least in the way his work juxtaposed individual experience with social meanings. Carl Jung had written of changing personal agendas as one moved closer to death, indeed a chapter by Jung was included in Feifal's ground-breaking book.

Of the existentialists, Victor Frankl (1962) was one of the most relevant. He writes that if there is no way out of suffering then we have a responsibility for the attitude in which we suffer. No one can tell another person what the meaning of his life should be. What people need is the time and opportunity to find their own meaning.

A sense of the spiritual, the psychological and the existential is to be found in the work of Elisabeth Kübler-Ross. She was critical of the Cartesian separation of mind and body and promoted a holistic consideration of the needs of dying people, including the need to help them find a meaning in their living and in their dying (Kübler-Ross 1969). But the therapeutic discourse of Kübler-Ross's holism is susceptible to the same risks as hospice care, that is, the shift to its becoming a technique rather than a philosophy. It may be that health care workers think they have achieved the aspired-to 'good death' if they can see the patient going through the Kübler-Ross stages. But to pursue a rigid prescriptive sequence devoid of spontaneity, flexibility or individuality is to reify technique to the exclusion of humanity (McNamara, Waddell & Colvin 1994).‡

SPIRITUAL PRACTICE AND SOCIAL CHANGE

I have considered the long tradition of spiritual care and the hospices and looked at a number of different factors impacting upon hospices in society. In so doing I have raised the question of how far a preoccupation with the *how* of hospice care has supplanted the *why* of its spiritual dimension. I have also looked at different ways of understanding death and dying.

A tradition of spiritual care had been exemplified by the work of religious institutions. These institutions and the assumptions they embodied about the relationship of the individual, society and the spiritual were being both criticized and supplanted by new ways of thinking about care. In this context the development of St Christopher's and then of the modern hospice movement both looked backwards in asserting the appropriateness of *spiritual* communities and looked forward in incorporating new understandings of the spiritual into their philosophy and practice.

A linking narrative in the spiritual, existential and sociological domains has been an engagement with the personal, with small-scale intimate experience. Alongside that has been a recognition of the shortcomings of grand narratives that seek to encompass all within themselves. In sociology this is a trend marked by postmodernism. In matters spiritual we see existentialism, mysticism and an engagement with the challenges of psychoanalysis. Paul Tillich and Martin Buber each make important contributions, revitalizing tradition and speaking directly about areas directly linked with the care of the dying. These were challenging ways forward of which Cicely Saunders and other pioneers of hospice care were well aware.

---

‡ A sense that Kübler-Ross' stages were the one true way and, as such, must be imposed on the recalcitrant dying is satirized in Bob Fosse's 1979 film *All that Jazz*.

Philip Reiff (1966) offered a view of society in which 'all creeds or none' were used in the systematic pursuit of the individual's sense of wellbeing, this was the 'triumph of the therapeutic'. He argues that

the professionally religious custodians of the old moral demands are no longer authoritative; although they still use languages of faith, that mode of moral communication that has lost its ties with either the controls or the remissions valid among their adherents; preaching, which once communicated revelatory messages, is a dead art, wrapping empty packages in elaborate solecisms. The preachers have little of either controlling or releasing functions and retain therefore little power seriously to affect or alter the emergent control system. It is in this sense that the Christian and Jewish professionals have lost their spiritual preceptorship. (Reiff 1966, p. 219)

But trenchant as these criticisms are, they could be outflanked by an approach that retained the spiritual while it did not seek to control; an approach that did not aspire to spiritual preceptorship in the hierarchical or institutional way Reiff identified. Indeed these alternative approaches colonized some of the language of what Reiff called the new 'anti-creed' of psychoanalysis. The emphasis was decidedly on the individual.

Paul Tillich described religion as the most fundamental aspect of the human spirit, the depth dimension of our shared humanity (Tillich 1988). Its essence is what he called 'ultimate concern', manifest in all creative functions of the human spirit (Tillich 1959). This ultimate concern is acted out in the many theatres of religious tradition but essentially in individual existence as a source of personal meaning, including at critical turning points like terminal illness and death (O'Connell 1995, p. 232).

Tillich saw (he was talking specifically about Americans before the Second World War) an anxiety about death which was met in two ways.

The reality of death is excluded from daily life to the highest possible degree. The dead are not allowed to show that they are dead; they are transformed into a mask of the living. The other and more important way of dealing with death is a belief in a continuation of life after death, called the immortality of the soul. (Tillich 1952, p. 111)

Tillich argues that the immortality of the soul is not a Christian ideal. Christianity speaks of resurrection and eternal life not immortality, time and world without end. The latter construes not eternal rest in God but 'an unlimited contribution to the dynamics of the universe'. It is akin to continuous participation in the production process.

The immortality of the soul is a poor symbol for the courage to be in the face of one's having to die. (Tillich 1952, p. 164)

Tillich's philosophy of health sees man as a multidimensional unity for whom healing always must include all dimensions (Tillich 1984). This is an approach in harmony with the hospice conceptualization of total care for total pain. But it is a holism that does not mean that one can collapse one dimension into another, for example by equating spiritual pain with some sort of psychological construct or by sidestepping an encounter with the transcendental.

Martin Buber's book *I and Thou* (1937) deals centrally with man's relationship with other men; it is concerned with social change and with the way one can differentiate the I–It relationship from the I–Thou only via reference to its ethical basis, the all embracing I–Thou relationship that is God (Bradshaw 1994, p. 295). His mysticism did not lead outside the world nor did it lead away from God.

Kaufmann guides our reading of Buber's *I and Thou* with the advice that we should open our hearts to hear what it has to say to us. When we do,

we are confronted with a crucial question: if God is to mean something to us, can it be anything but what Buber suggests ... namely the eternal Thou? All superstitions *about* God, all talk about him, all theology is sacrificed to the voice that speaks to us, the *Du* to which some cry out "when", as Goethe says, "man in his agony grows mute". And not only in agony.

Buber succeeds in endowing the social sphere with a religious dimension. Where other critics of religion tend to take away the sabbath and leave us with a life of weekdays, Buber attacks the dichotomy that condemns men to lives that are at least six-sevenths drab. ... The place of the sacred is not a house of God, no church, synagogue, or seminary, nor one day in seven, and the span of the sacred is much shorter than twenty-four hours. The sabbath is every day, several times a day. (Kaufmann 1970, p. 30)

These are approaches to the spiritual that resonate with the founding ideas of St Christopher's:

in His own way God would meet the patient if he was allowed to. The role of the hospice was somehow to hold the door open. (Saunders 1987)

Everyone could be involved in the spiritual:

Disease is a sombre mystery, a powerful transformative process that leads to the gateways of death. Both physician and the religious specialist have much concern with this boundary between life and death and those who are specially effective at their callings traverse with respectful familiarity along this distinctive edge. (Birnbaum 1989, p. 33)

THE YALE COLLOQUIUM

Although there had been close links between the emerging thinking about hospice care in the UK and the developing provision in the USA, not least through personnel involvement of Dame Cicely and others from St Christopher's, there was a sense, identified by US hospice pioneer Florence Wald, that there existed a 'basic flaw in our perception of hospice care from the beginning. Cicely Saunders' blend of medical science and spiritual care wasn't appreciated by many of us' (Wald 1986: 25). The result was that the spiritual side of the care of the terminally ill had not, in Wald's view, been developed in the USA. In 1986 she convened a colloquium in Yale in an attempt to address how, in that context, the spiritual could be reincorporated. Its deliberations illustrate the way the spiritual sits alongside other discourses in the development of care for the terminally ill.

While the participants in Yale explored humanist, Judaic and Buddhist assumptions and considered the nuances of the term 'spiritual' there was at the Colloquium's heart a difference of approach that such a broad ecumenical, not to say eclectic, approach could not reconcile. In effect, for some people, one could not get rid of God and still meaningfully explore the spiritual. The Christian chaplain Carleton Sweetser argues that it is the resurrection that is the cornerstone of hospice care:

For this writer it is difficult to conceive of spiritual issues of death and dying as unrelated to religious faith, unrelated to an objective deity at work in the world and in the affairs of human beings through the spirit. (Sweetser 1986, p. 112)

Samuel Klagsbrun, talking about his Judaism, said

Spirituality cannot be separated from its source, which is the revealed God. (Klagsbrun 1986, p. 78)

Dame Cicely, writing to Florence Wald about the Yale Colloquium, tells her that 'I think we have to stop bending over backwards not to upset the secular group' (in Wald 1986: 161). It is as if, by the mid 1980s, the alliance of backgrounds and attitudes that made up the hospice movement had become both disparate and fragile to the extent that one had to appease those who found talking of the spiritual difficult. This was done by adopting a language which missed out God. But in so doing one lost a language of faith, vocation, mystery and the permission of those whose understanding was intrinsically linked with Christian service and resurrection to define their work using these terms. Everyone ended up speaking the language of psychology.§

A SPIRITUAL TRADITION WITHOUT GOD?

While it is often the case that spiritual is equated with religiosity (Stifoss-Hanssen & Kallenberg 1996, p. 21) there have also been thoughtful attempts to seek a definition that locates the spiritual with

the transcendental, inspirational, and existential way to live one's life as well as, in a fundamental and profound sense, with the person as a human being. (IWG 1994, p. 33)

While such a definition might placate those who feel uncomfortable with the spiritual/religious formulation, it is an attempt at eclecticism that also risks loosing both the modesty and the poetics of a numinous spirituality. It is the encounter with the deity that allows one to put oneself in the hands of something greater than oneself. Without that there is a danger that a reliance on the self can fall short of what one needs at the end of life.

Something of those shortcomings are evident in survey results from North America: 94% of American hospice programmes failed to demonstrate adequate spiritual care when surveyed. Only 5% of Canadian hospice programmes have a chaplain as part of the team (Ley 1992). But the shortcomings can also be approached via further contemplating what is put in place when the spiritual and the religious are separated. Seale (1995), in talking of death in late modern society, identifies how we can now proclaim a heroic self-identity in the face of death and we can do this via gaining knowledge and demonstrating courage. It is a demanding and lonely possibility. MacIntyre (1985) sees a shift from a society with supposed fixed and accepted universal moral norms to one where values rest in whatever methods and techniques produce psychological effectiveness. This is a 'morals' of expediency approach that can also feel that one is cast adrift. In the context of hospices Bradshaw (1996) incisively sums up a shift from the 'power of the soul' to 'soul-less power'.

---

§ In spring 1996, as part of the Wellcome History of Medicine funded Hospice History Project, I visited the USA where I met and interviewed Florence Wald, Carleton Sweetser and Samuel Klagsbrun. The nature of the spiritual in hospice care was one of many subjects we considered. It is my intention to report more fully on their contributions, and those of others in the USA, in future work.

CONCLUSION

In this chapter I have identified a tradition of spiritual care in hospices and have looked at the way hospice practice sits comfortably with a new direction in that tradition. This is the direction that accepts the insights of Frankl and others in recognizing that the key to spiritual care for the dying is not in having answers but in being there. I have considered influences other than the spiritual on the way hospices practise and have sought to underline a danger in both unduly elevating technique and also in thinking that one has to seek a lowest common denominator agreement in order include the spiritual in total care.

I have looked at ways of conceptualizing the spiritual without God. These concepts contain shortcomings both for people at the end of their lives and for those who care for them. They also have shortcomings for Christians who, in the interests of a new triumphant psychology and of not offending others, are being asked to remain quiet about their vocation and their belief in the resurrection, the very things that carry with them the strength needed at the end of a person's life.

Hospices have a place in the overall health care system greater than their physical size. That place is to maintain and promote interdisciplinary total care for total pain. They do impact outside their own narrow realm of practice. But there is impact both ways. Hospices have been, and are increasingly being, subjected to the influences and pressures other forms of health care are under. A danger is that the example they offer will be dissipated. What they have specifically to offer will be less clearly differentiated from the systems they could influence.

One area where they have built on the traditions of hospice through the centuries is that of spiritual care. But this is not immune from being compromised. Pressures come from within — a wish to be sensitive to difference — and from without — a pervasive psychology and an accompanying elevation of technique. But within hospices some have engaged with a new spirituality, one that does not feel the need to sideline God, and one that can still celebrate individuality and the search for meaning.

At the level of the social, James poses a fascinating question when she asks:

While hospices have achieved much, the Voluntary Euthanasia Society has 11,000 members in Britain and the numbers are growing. It will be interesting to see how history interprets the morality of a society in which two contrasting groups, each with deeply committed views on human dignity, develop in parallel. (James 1994, p. 125)

But the challenge this question presents might be addressed by wondering if we can, any longer, speak of the morality of society. If we cannot, then we must engage with the morality of my contact with you and the authenticity, and for some of us the spirituality, of care.

The absence of clarity in terms of social constructions of the moral and the need to devise a spiritual response that incorporates both the individual's search for meaning and the presence of God presents both a challenge and an opportunity for the developing tradition of spiritual care in hospices.

REFERENCES

Ahmedzai S 1993 The medicalization of dying: a doctor's view. In: Clark D (ed) The future for palliative care. Open University Press, Buckingham

Birnbaum R 1989 Chinese Buddhist traditions of healing and the life cycle. In: Sullivan L E (ed) Healing and restoring: health and medicine in the world's religious traditions. Macmillan, New York pp 33–57

Biswas B 1993 The medicalization of dying: a nurse's view. In: Clark D (ed) The future for palliative care. Open University Press, Buckingham

Bradshaw A 1994 Lighting the lamp. Scutari Press, Harrow

Bradshaw A 1996 The spiritual dimension of hospice: the secularisation of an ideal. Social Science and Medicine 43(2): 409–419

Buber M 1937 I and thou. T & T Clark, Edinburgh

Davie G 1994 Religion in Britain since 1945. Blackwell, London

Dix A 1996 Is God good value? Health Service Journal, 11 July: 24–27

Feifal H 1959 The meaning of death. McGraw-Hill, New York

Frankl V 1962 Man's search for meaning: an introduction to logotherapy. Beacon Press, Boston

Froggatt K A, Walter T 1995 Hospice logos. Journal of Palliative Care 11(4): 39–47

HMSO 1989 Working for patients. HMSO, London

International Work Group on Death, Dying and Bereavement (IWG) 1994 Assumptions and principles of spiritual care. In: Corr C A, Morgan J D, Wass H Statements on death, dying and bereavement. London, Ontario

James N 1994 From vision to system: the maturing of the hospice movement. In: Lee R, Morgan D (eds) Death rites: law and ethics at the end of life. Routledge, London

James N, Field D 1992 The routinisation of hospice: charisma and bureaucratisation. Social Science and Medicine 34(2): 1363–1375

Johnson I, Rogers C, Biswas B, Ahmedzai S 1990 What do hospices do? A survey of hospices in the United Kingdom and Republic of Ireland. British Medical Journal 300 (24 March): 791–793

Johnston-Taylor E, Amenta M, Highfield M 1995 A comparison of oncology and hospice nurses's spiritual care perspectives and practices. Oncology Nursing Forum 22(2): 352

Kaufmann W 1970 I and thou: a prologue. In: Buber M I and thou, 3rd edn. T & T Clark, Edinburgh

Klagsbrun S 1986 Spiritual help from Judaic and psychiatric perspectives. In: Wald, op cit.

Kübler-Ross E 1970 On death and dying. Routledge, London
Lamerton R 1980 Care of the dying. Penguin, Harmondsworth
Ley D 1992 Spiritual care in hospice. In: Cox G R, Fundis R J (eds) Spiritual, ethical and pastoral aspects of death and bereavement. Baywood Publishing, Amityville, NY
MacIntyre A 1985 After virtue. Duckworth, London
McNamara B, Waddell C, Colvin M 1994 The institutionalisation of the good death. Social Science and Medicine. 39(11): 1501–1508
Mitchell B 1994 Faith and criticism. Clarendon Press, Oxford
NAHAT 1997 Spiritual care in the NHS: a guide for purchasers and providers. National Association of Health Authorities and Trusts, London
O'Connell L J 1995 Religious dimensions of dying and death. Western Journal of Medicine 163: 231–235
Penson J, Fisher R 1991 Palliative care for people with cancer. Edward Arnold, Leeds
Reiff P 1966 The triumph of the therapeutic. Penguin, Harmondsworth
Saunders C 1965 Watch with me. Nursing Times, 26 November: 1–3
Saunders C 1987 I was sick and you visited me. Christian Nurse International 3: 4–5
Saunders C 1996 A personal therapeutic journey. British Medical Journal 313: 1599–1601
Seale C 1995 Heroic death. Sociology 29(4): 597–613
St Christopher's Hospice 1988 Statement of Foundation Group aim and basis. London
Stifoss-Hanssen H, Kallenberg K 1996 Existential questions and health. Swedish Council for Planning and Coordination of Research, Stockholm
Sweetser C 1986 Hospice care and faith: a Christian perspective. In: Wald, op cit
Tillich P 1952 The courage to be. Fontana, London
Tillich P 1959 Theology of culture. Oxford University Press, Oxford
Tillich P 1984 The meaning of health: essays in existentialism, psychoanalysis and religion. Exploration Press, Chicago
Tillich P 1988 The relationship today between science and religion. In: Thomas J M (ed) The spiritual situation in our technical society. Mercer University Press, Macon
Titmuss R 1970 The gift relationship. George Allen & Unwin, London
Torrens P 1981 Achievement, failure and the future: hospice analysed. In: Saunders C, Summers D H, Teller N (eds) Hospice: the living idea. Edward Arnold, London
Wald F 1986 In quest of the spiritual component of care for the terminally ill. Yale University School of Nursing, New Haven
Walter T 1997 The ideology and organization of spiritual care: three approaches. Palliative Medicine 11: 21–30
Weber M 1976 The Protestant ethic and the spirit of capitalism. George Allen & Unwin, London

Spiritual values in a secular age

Janet Bellamy

INTRODUCTION

In 1977 a UK Department of Education and Science document on the curriculum included the statement, '"Spiritual" is a meaningless adjective for the atheist and of dubious use to the agnostic' (Priestley 1996). 'Spiritual' is thus seen as coterminous with religious, and because it is assumed that we live in an increasingly secular or non-religious society, the assumption is that we have 'come of age' and no longer need concepts of spirituality. Such a reductionist view needs to be challenged.

The secular world in which we live is based on particular ideals, meanings and aspirations which are themselves reflections of spiritual values. It is a world, it will be argued, which values technological progress, free enterprise, competition, profit, individualism and change. These values have been expressed in ways which have distorted or destroyed many traditional social and economic structures and assumptions. Unemployment, an increasing gap between rich and poor (on both a global and national level), the fragmentation of communities and environmental devastation are perceived as the inevitable costs of such developments; problems to be managed in order that the ideals of the new era can be safeguarded and pursued. A growing sense of alienation and meaninglessness among the dispossessed can be discerned in the abuse of drugs and alcohol, the abrogation of democratic processes, the increasing suicide rate and the violence of attacks upon others, from the unprovoked muggings of the elderly to the horrors of genocide.

At the same time, however, alternative spiritual values are discernible. They are expressed in both traditional and contemporary forms and they provide a focus of hope and new meaning. It is our contemporary secular society, for example, which is beginning to recognize the injustice of deeply rooted discrimination and prejudice on such grounds as race, gender, sexuality, disability and class and thus to challenge the traditional spiritual values which supported patriarchy, privilege and possession.

It is thus naïve to assume that contemporary ideologies are responsible for the end of a golden age of spiritual values. Similarly, it is simplistic to assume that spiritual values are of necessity good; they can be powerfully destructive.

This chapter will examine the following four themes which appear to illustrate key contemporary values:

- the mechanistic problem-solving approach
- individualism
- dualism
- the asymmetric nature of relationships.

It will attempt to show how they are reflected not only in current attitudes to British health care but also in a wider context. In addition it will attempt to identify signs of hope and possibilities of adaptation and change to a more holistic and creative agenda. First, however, it is necessary to explore the concept of spirituality more fully.

WHAT ARE SPIRITUAL VALUES?

The dust jacket of *A Dictionary of Christian Spirituality* (Wakefield 1983) defines spirituality as a term, 'used widely to describe that inner sense of searching for God, which, in many different forms, not all of them specifically religious, is part of human make-up even in today's secular world'. Like the title of this chapter, this statement provides an explicit indication of the ambiguity of the meanings implied by the terms spiritual, religious and secular and of their interrelationships.

Some of the ambiguity reflects changing conceptual frameworks. As Cupitt (1988) points out, 'linguistic meanings are relative, differential and historically changing'. Recently, spiritual has come to be understood as a broader and more diffuse term than religious, including and giving meaning to that which is secular or non-religious as well as to the religious. Spiritual can be seen as that which integrates the psychosocial and biological, a means of assessing, evaluating and interpreting the experience of life. It may or it may not include an understanding of transcendence. Since the Enlightenment, existentialism, pragmatism, crude logical positivism and relativism have worked together to question the old concept of God on which so much of the language of both religious and spiritual writings is based. It is not necessary to accept traditional ways of conceptualizing spirituality in order to accept its existence. There is an important distinction, for example, between belief in a transcendent God and an understanding of ultimate values in human life. Both express spirituality; only the first is couched in religious language.

Thus the term 'spiritual' can be said to concern three main aspects of human experience:

- Values; that which is valued and the way in which it is valued.
- Meaning; the quest for life-enhancing meaning which does not preclude mystery but which does not necessitate looking for a supernatural factor.
- Relatedness; the human need to find self-worth and identity, to love and be loved, to be accepted or forgiven. This relatedness may involve the self, other people, the environment, the transcendent.

Spiritual values may therefore be found in secular and in religious societies. It is important to recognize, however, that attempts to define spirituality are not only fraught with difficulty but also with danger. Definition is a tool of rationality, an instrument which seeks to enclose. The term spiritual, however, needs to remain elusive if it is not to betray its very identity; inherent to it is the concept of searching rather than finding. If Cupitt is right in his assertion that we make truth and we make values, it seems vital that all are aware of the importance of their endeavour and the limitations of their perspective. This was recognized by T.S. Eliot writing in 1928:

Where is the wisdom we have lost in knowledge?
Where is the knowledge we have lost in information?

(The Rock)

In an attempt to discover what is creative and what is destructive in contemporary values, we turn first to the mechanistic problem-solving approach.

THE MECHANISTIC PROBLEM-SOLVING APPROACH

The influence of this value in modern life is pervasive and profound. In the laudable quest for answers to questions, the desire for answers has often ignored the effects of the means of discovery; the need to arrive at the destination has destroyed the value and meaning of the journey. New technology both reflects and creates this approach. Computers provide instant communication based on unassailably logical systems; it is, however, a form of communication which changes the way people relate to each other. Fax machines and e-mail reduce the need to speak to others. New retail programmes aim to render 'going shopping' anachronistic. Educators are encouraged to produce distance learning packages to obviate interpersonal dynamics in the learning process. Meanwhile, concepts such as spirituality which fit uneasily into a world of rational discourse become part of a school curriculum which is no longer 'hidden' but invisible.

This model thus reflects the value and meaning attributed to problem solving and to mechanisms and systems as a means of achieving it. If people are involved in the systems, they are regarded as subordinate to them. Thus personnel officers are now known as human resource managers. Organizations are increasingly hierarchical. There has been a burgeoning of management theory and an explosion of institutional turbulence. Despite the flimsiness of the ideas on which it is based, current management practice often assumes it is undergirded by an absolute truth, buttressed by its new language of mission statements, goal setting, outcome measurement, performance-related pay, down-sizing and rationalization. A recent article outlined the possibilities of 'evolution-based management'. Charlton (1996) argues that 'according to evolutionary psychology the human mind is a collection of specialised mechanisms each designed by natural selection to solve a problem of survival'. By tapping into this innate psychology, it is thought, bureaucratic substitutes can be minimized and effective management achieved. Here, then, is demonstrated the mechanistic problem-solving approach, and we should note its dangers. 'Change management presupposes that the future can be predicted and controlled; utilitarian philosophers know to their embarrassment that the consequences of actions may be very unpredictable indeed' (Pattison 1995). In all this the human beings at the heart of the process are seen as means to an end.

How is this model reflected in health care? Even before change management theories were imposed with such devastating human consequences on the National Health Service, the mechanistic problem-solving approach was well established. The Western medical model is powerfully entrenched not only in the West but also, with tragic consequences, in the two-thirds world. It is hierarchical, based on scientific methods of diagnosis and treatment. 'Diseases' are classified, norms established and there is a reliance on the efficacy of surgery or drug therapy to 'cut out' or destroy. The authority of doctors is unquestioned.

The pervasive influence of the medical model can be seen in the 'deliverance' model of nursing care developed since the 1970s. The nursing process is based on the interpretation of need, planning of goals and priorities, identification of steps to implement them and evaluation and reassessment of effects. Attempts to transfer this process to the assessment of spiritual need and delivery of spiritual care has been discussed earlier in this book. There is a dangerous assumption that spirituality can be classified and controlled, quantified and processed in such a way that questions about ultimate values and intimate areas of relationship can be asked and recorded in the same way as questions about fluid balances, bowel function and body chemistry.

A major difficulty is that the medical model has provided a method which has defeated the principle on which its endeavour originated. The desire to restore life has tended to subordinate quality to quantity. The desire to give spiritual care arose from this. It reflects awareness of the need for holistic care based on a recognition of the patient not as the intestinal obstruction in the third bed but as one with a unique identity and response to hospitalization. If, however, there is too much emphasis on the subdivision of that person into the physical, psychological, social and spiritual aspects, each with their own subdivisions to be evaluated and classified, the result so fragments and distorts reality that the concepts of holism and uniqueness are lost. Herein lies the dilemma, for the alternatives to this approach seem either too amorphous and unfocused or else reduced to specific religious or cultural needs.

A parallel can be found in the development of counselling theory and practice. The significance of psychological needs is increasingly recognized but the assessment and meeting of these needs is being forced into the same mechanistic problem-solving approach. Teams of counsellors are rushed in to disaster areas as if their very presence will solve the 'problems' of the tragedy of sudden death and destruction. GP surgeries are adding counsellors to their primary health care teams, often with unhelpful assumptions about the counsellor's ability to teach patients to 'manage' their anxiety or bereavement problems in as short a time as possible. Similarly, the rapid growth of Employee Assistance Programmes providing counselling for workers reflects the employer's desire for a 'quick fix'. Counsellors are required to be skilled in brief therapy and to work within an externally imposed time-limited framework. A plethora of paperwork whereby needs are assessed, goals identified and achievement monitored confirm the adherence to a mechanistic medical model. Meanwhile there is widespread interest in a new counselling method, solution-focused therapy. Its nomenclature is significant; Rogerian person-centred concepts are unable to meet the demand for speed and quantifiable results.

One reason for the inadequacy of the mechanistic approach lies in its reliance on linear thinking. Its emphasis on problems and solutions, giver to receiver, meaninglessness to meaning reveals an oversimplistic, two-dimensional mode of thought which distorts reality. This easily becomes reductionist thinking. Analysing theories of depression, Bringle (1996) illustrates how the biological reductionist asks for a pill, the spiritual reductionist seeks a sin for which she is being punished, the sociopolitical reductionist blames the oppressive society in which she lives, and the sociopsychological reductionist recognizes the interaction of destructive relationship scripts of past and present. 'Single strands are simpler to unravel than whole tapestries and tangles ... simplicity is seductively appealing.' Tapestries are based on the interweaving of straight lines; it is their interrelationship which creates both the pattern and the strength of the whole. Feminists provide an alternative to linear thinking. Women's experience, it is argued, is cyclical. Growth is spiral not linear. Relationships grow in a circle of loving and being loved, of returning to one's own inner places and moving from inside out again. Herein perhaps lies the tangle which is the reality of human experience.

Another reason for the inadequacy of the mechanistic approach is its emphasis on 'needs'. This creates a problem-solving orientation and reflects what Walter (1985) argues is a fashionable perception of the self as a collection of needs, the meeting of which has, he argues, replaced traditional spiritual values in the directing of our lives. 'Thus Descartes' "I think therefore I am", has been replaced by the philosophy "I need therefore I am".' Love, Walter claims, has been reconceived in terms of bureaucratized welfare in which the person is a bundle of needs allocated to particular professions who are in business to meet them. Nursing literature on spiritual care frequently cites Maslow's hierarchy of needs. Maslow (1970) proclaimed that he was committed to an 'attempt to do what the formal religions have tried to do and failed to do, that is to offer people an understanding of human nature, a frame of reference in which they could understand when they ought to feel guilty and when they ought not to feel guilty … we are working up what amounts to a scientific ethics'. Here is the mechanistic problem-solving approach par excellence, clearly organized, hierarchical and capable of evaluation and delivery. It reflects an achievement-oriented individualistic capitalistic society. It is essential to respect and avoid the dangers in such an uncritical and oversimplified view of human nature.

Schumacher (1974) was right to point out that 'the cultivation and expansion of needs is the antithesis of wisdom'. Similarly the cultivation and expansion of a mechanistic problem-solving approach is the antithesis of a creative spirituality. This does not mean an iconoclastic destruction of all linear thinking and systematized knowledge and structures. It means appraising its process and consequences more critically, being aware of the multidimensional effects on relationships made by the tapestry's interaction of warp on weft and so empowering people instead of delivering decontextualized solutions. It means revisiting another of the pervasive values which underlies contemporary society: individualism.

INDIVIDUALISM

In Britain the individualism of the 1960s has developed into the consumerism of the 1990s. We have been encouraged to become self-sufficient and to strive for self-fulfilment and self-actualization. The growth of a strong central state denigrates the concept of society and obviates the need for corporate responsibility. To take account of the needs of those who fail to realize their individual potential is seen at best in terms of moral duty or at worst as political expediency; success is judged in terms of the lowest cost necessary to achieve it. Inherent in this individualism is a fragmentation influenced by the reductionism discussed above. Individuals and societies alike are subdivided into constituent parts. Health is perceived narrowly, its links with its socioeconomic and political context ignored.

The flourishing of counselling and psychotherapy is an example of the appeal of individualism. The individual deliberately takes herself out of her normal support mechanisms and seeks another individual who is and will continue to be a stranger to her. It is perhaps significant that the world of counselling and psychotherapy is characterized by fragmentation. The burgeoning of books on spirituality reflect a similarly individualistic emphasis, often reducing it to private peace of mind techniques. In the nursing literature, although spirituality is seen in terms of relationship, spiritual care is seen almost exclusively in terms of an individual nurse giving care to an individual patient through a relationship of trust in her. There is a silence about the corporate nature of spirituality in a hospital ward or the spirituality of the institution as a whole.

The organization of professions within health care also reflects this fragmentation. Hospital staff, for example, form a complex and fragmented group of parallel hierarchies whose ability to communicate with each other is often poor and lacks mutual respect. Lip service is paid to multidisciplinary approaches; often, however, these create additional defensive barriers and stress.

Meanwhile NHS reforms mean the creation of separate rival trusts each of which to survive and prosper has sought to expand its sphere of influence. Homogeneity of purpose is no longer a requirement; competition among purchasers is encouraged. Such rampant consumerism not only fails to meet the needs of the people who are the least influential and for whom the NHS was originally created but also, in the spiral of costs it engenders, helps to increase the financial problems which threaten to dismember it altogether.

Individualism and fragmentation are reflected in government policies as a whole. Health, social services, employment and economic agencies, for example, are seen as independent of each other, competing for funds. Hart's 'inverse care law' of 1971, that social inequalities are negatively correlated with health has been ignored. The so-called 'Black Report', *Inequalities in Health*, of 1980 pointed out that bringing all adults aged between 16 and 64 up to the mortality experience of social class 1 would mean 39 000 fewer deaths a year. Research by the Rowntree Foundation and Public Health Alliance continues to show the links between wealth and health: that inequalities are reflected in differential morbidity and mortality figures. Individualism, however, means that while the rich in class 1 are encouraged to buy private health insurance, the poor continue to visit the GP with, for example, chronic respiratory problems. The GP cannot change their housing yet it is estimated by Friends of the Earth that tackling cold and damp housing could save the NHS a thousand million pounds a year. Similarly, the GP is not able to prescribe the means to buy an adequate diet. The disappearance of markets and cheap corner shops has militated against the poor; a poor diet contributes to ill-health. Meanwhile, fund-holding practices provide quicker hospital care for their patients; fund-holding is less common in inner cities where poverty is concentrated. The

Child Poverty Action Group revealed in 1996 that while average incomes in Britain rose 37% between 1979 and 1993, the poorest section of the population experienced a fall of 18%. Since 1979 there has been a threefold increase in people living in poverty. The report called for stronger employment rights, more flexible benefits and a more progressive taxation structure. All those remedies would mean eroding the individualistic emphasis of self-interest and a competitive free market. Attempts to provide health care will continue to founder while it is seen in a narrowing medical context, separated in concept and funding from its essential concomitants. Health will continue to be elusive while the goal of equity is replaced by the goal of economy. Those who cannot compete effectively, such as the elderly, the poor and the chronic sick, will continue to bear the cost disproportionately. This was foreseen in 1991: 'health care will come to be viewed more as a privilege than as a right and reforms will prove to be less of an answer to an economic crisis and more the provoking of a moral crisis' (Bellamy & Pike 1991).

What, then, are the alternatives to individualism? To recognize and celebrate the individuality of personhood is life-giving and not to be destroyed or despised. It must, however, be balanced and contextualized. Just as a baby knows its mother before it knows itself, so sociality is as important as individuality. It was Frankl, a survivor of the holocaust, who pointed out that human existence is essentially self-transcendence rather than self-actualization. The major religions reflect a corporate not individualistic view of humanity. In Judaism, Christianity and in Islam, for example, spiritual values are inextricably bound up with social justice, and it is this which has been lost in the quest for individualism. It is vital to provide a care for individuals which does not consign their context to effective oblivion. There must be an assessment of the injustices, inequalities and dehumanizing influences of the environment.

'Spiritual well-being is the affirmation of life in a relationship with God, self, community and environment that nurtures and celebrates wholeness' (Moberg 1979). This aim was reflected in the publication by the World Health Organization (WHO) of *Health for All 2000* in 1988. Based on the seminal work of the Alma Ata conference a decade earlier, its aim was to remove the inequities caused by the Western medical model and to improve the overall quality of life for individuals and communities through their own active involvement and participation. Of central concern was poverty; 'to improve the health of any society', asserted Mahler in his address to the Assembly, 'it is necessary to raise the level of health of its least privileged members. This is not only an epidemiological truism, it is a moral obligation'.

Britain continues to subscribe to the WHO ideals, and there are occasional signs of attempts to put them into practice. In 1996, for example, the Public Health Trust received grants to develop a public health approach to primary care. This means going beyond the individual patient or family to the community in which they live and taking account of the social and economic environment. Meanwhile, educationalists are advocating reform of the dominant biomedical content of medical education and the integration of social, preventive, economic and ethical aspects of medicine to provide a greater understanding of contextual issues. Such efforts are yet to be broadly realized; there is, however, hope in the attempt. One of the obstacles to integration, however, lies in the third contemporary value to be examined, that of dualism.

DUALISM

Dualism is characterized by an oversimplification and polarizing of issues. Reality is seen as comprising two distinct entities. Things are thus conceptualized as problems and solutions, good and bad, right and wrong, physical and psychological, material and spiritual, individual or corporate, living or dead. There is nothing new in this approach nor in its harmful effects. Fundamentalist religions and political ideologies throughout history have attempted to impose harsh dualistic concepts on others. Such ideas flourish in times of insecurity and turmoil; it is significant that there is an upsurge of fundamentalism at the present time. Fundamentalists have an unassailable belief in their own rectitude. Often this implies a need to root out and destroy what is regarded as wrong or evil.

Recent health care reforms illustrate the effects of dualism. The solution to growing financial problems was identified as a far-reaching structural change whereby purchasers and providers of health care were separated. This dualistic solution quickly acquired the status of absolute truth, although it remains little more than a costly act of faith.

The medical model is itself dualistic, encompassing a polarity between cure and care. Doctors traditionally have been seen as superior, the authors of cure, while nurses have been seen as inferior, the givers of care. Hospitals are seen as providers of life. Death is seen as failure, to be camouflaged, minimized or avoided. Hospitals are seen as temples of cure; the more advanced the technical and scientific methodology, the more prestigious the institution. Caring for the dying thus became the preserve of a new institution, the hospice, largely dependent on voluntary funding. The concept of hospices providing new insights to be integrated into hospital care and thus rendering themselves redundant has itself died; indeed the hospice movement is in danger of creating its own prestigious ethos. The aim to provide a 'good' death, for example, is in danger of overriding the complexity of the reality of people's experience of dying. Disabled people also have experienced the destructive effects of dualism, having been seen as 'either tragic victims needing compassion or triumphant heroes inviting emulation' (Pattison 1994).

What are the alternatives? Change in the values of government is required. British government is based on anachronistic and destructive processes. Not only is good government hindered by the fragmentation of departmentalism discussed above but also by the ritualized, polarized conduct of political debate. 'The importance of renewing democracy in Britain stems not only from its intrinsic benefits ... but from its instrumental value in achieving sustainability and social justice' argues the Real World Coalition (1996). There needs to be much more emphasis on the environmental crisis, the changes in the global economic order and the implications worldwide of rising inequality and decreasing social cohesion. Market forces need to be the servants not the leaders of policy decisions. There needs to be commitment to social justice and a new integrated relationship between individual and corporate needs. An integrated system of planning requires public accountability and commitment which in turn is dependent upon a high quality of education and media communication.

In health provision, holistic care which takes account of the context from which the person comes, needs to replace the philosophy of cure at all cost. The hierarchical mechanistic medical model with its compartmentalized approach to patient 'management' and the perpetuation of a circumscribed 'sick role' needs to be modified.

A bridge is thus needed between those whose work and vision is in the broad political and social realm and those whose work is with the individual, for, in separating the two, another form of dualism is created. To be committed to justice and to be in solidarity with the vulnerable does not belong exclusively to either reality. Pattison argues that counsellors, for example, who represent an individualistic perspective should seek to identify oppression and alienation within the social structures of their clients, should eschew the reductionism and stereotyping which invalidates a just social order and reflect upon the social and political significance of their own practice and activity. 'Individualist diagnoses and solutions are not adequate. Are we willing to hear the dull thump of the poor knocking on the consulting room door and so inconveniently disturbing the calm of the therapeutic conversation?' (Pattison 1991). It is not only counsellors of whom that question must be asked, but all who work with individuals. Similarly, those whose influence is in the broader sphere must ask searching questions of the effects of their work on individuals who do not neatly fit the 'norms' ascribed to them. The key to this may lie partly in in modifying the asymmetric nature of both personal and global relationships.

THE ASYMMETRIC NATURE OF RELATIONSHIPS

Attention has already been drawn to the increasing differentials between governments and the governed, rich and poor, the powerful and the powerless.

To feel depressed, cheated, bitter, desperate, vulnerable, frightened, angry, worried about debts or job and housing insecurity; to feel devalued, useless, helpless, uncared for, hopeless, isolated, anxious and a failure: these feelings can dominate people's whole experience of life, colouring their experience of everything else. It is the chronic stress arising from feelings like these which does the damage. (Wilkinson 1996)

In global terms the belief that Free Trade is beneficial to all has driven regional trade agreements and International Monetary Fund (IMF) aid to developing countries. Debt repayments often exceed what is spent on health and education within those countries, and the links between poverty, economic degradation and poor health and the power imbalance between the so-called 'first' world and the 'two-thirds' world are more firmly forged.

In terms of British health care, the asymmetric nature of relationships is reflected in the language of codes of practice and professional literature. An active interventionist approach is encouraged. Health workers must promote, prevent, restore, deliver and 'manage' their care. Thus both cure and care are objectified, delivered from the powerful to the powerless. The continuing use of the term patient, with its root in passivity and its link with notions of tolerance, is significant. A new word has just been coined by psychotherapists to combine 'patient' and 'client'; the choice of 'plient', with its obvious links to pliancy, is further evidence of deeply rooted asymmetry.

Asymmetric relationships characterize health service organization. The *Health Service Journal* is full of references to the increasing number of internal disputes, bitter feuds and dramatic resignations and sackings in and between the new trusts. Rising workloads, staff shortages, job insecurity and autocratic organizations are all contributing to higher levels of stress in the NHS (Moore 1996). Staff mental health was found to be nearly twice as good in trusts with greater cooperation, better communications and participatory decision-making processes; that this needs to be rediscovered is a sad and significant reflection of the destructive effects of new management styles. A powerful critique of 'modern' management's quasi-religious, self-authenticating monolithic style is provided by Pattison (1997).

What are the alternatives to these inhumane relationships? Koestler was told 'you have the vanity to give but you lack the generosity to take'. In giving, we are in a position of strength, able to dictate our terms and bask in the glow of virtue of power. This, as has been shown, can be destructive and dehumanizing. To receive, however, requires generosity and insight; the generosity to relinquish control of the relationship and to take what is offered, and the insight to recognize the motivation of the donor and the nature of the gift. Asymmetric relationships depend on the dualism of giver *or* receiver; they are based on a fear of receiving, a fear of vulnerability expressed as a determination to control.

A more healthy and helpful relationship lies in what Rumbold (1986) describes as 'asymmetric mutuality'. This takes account of the role difference without removing the element of mutuality which converts the relationship into one of I–Thou instead of subject and object. That is possible only when the vulnerability of the helper, the one in whom power is invested, is acknowledged by both. Modern pastoral theology reflects this in terms of Nouwen's 'wounded healer' whose acknowledgement of weakness and vulnerability becomes a source of healing (1972). The professional dispenser of cure or care is defending herself from that possibility.

Signs of hope exist that changes are occurring. Anita Roddick's New Academy of Business attempts to address the inhumanity of the current business ethic. Four main targets have been identified: social justice (especially the effects of global trade on partners in developing countries), sustainability, corporate citizenship and the 'enlightened' workplace (whereby the needs of workers are accorded importance). These concepts are reflected in Professor West's recommendations for reducing worker stress in the NHS. He suggests that multiple and radical change is required, including a reduction in workload, an increasing sense of staff control and improved teamwork. Individual patient care reflects the benefits of asymmetric mutuality when staff have the courage to remove professional masks and permit patients to determine the quantity and quality of help given without a defensive or stereotypical response.

CONCLUSION

It is no good asking what is the meaning of life because life isn't the answer, life is the question, and you are the answer. (Le Guin, 1988).

Herein, perhaps, lies the key in any search for spiritual values. If we accept a concept of humanity as a creation in process, it follows that spiritual values are not given but discovered. Whether the society in which we live is regarded as secular or religious, it is important that the process of discovery is open to all both as beneficiaries and as participants. It is a process which needs to eschew reductionism and dualism and be fired by a desire to go beyond what is recognized as provisional. It needs to understand the vulnerability and fragmentariness of human experience not as a threat but as a promise of a life-giving mutuality. It is a process which needs to encompass the uniqueness of the individual within a context of social and political justice. Justice requires concepts of community which cross the boundaries imposed by race, gender, disability, class, nationality, sexuality, age and belief systems. To achieve this, many traditional values have been questioned and found wanting. This, too, is part of the process. Our fear of vulnerability and uncertainty leads us to seek security in authoritarian absolutes whose simplicity often distorts reality and gives false hope. Experience helps us to distinguish between the values which are creative and those which are destructive; it is an experience, however, which must be lived in community and not in isolation. Perhaps, like justice and truth, spirituality is a concept which can never be completely grasped. Incompleteness should not deter us from the search, just as the impossibility of finding answers should not deter us from asking questions. It is, however, important to remember the complexity, the sensitivity and the vulnerability of the human beings who provide the focus of the quest.

REFERENCES

Bellamy P, Pyke L 1991 Health for all and the NHS reforms. Contact 104: 21–24
Black D, Morris J, Smith C, Townsend P 1980 Inequalities in health. Penguin, London
Bringle M 1996 Soul-dye and salt: integrating spiritual and medical understandings of depression. Journal of Pastoral Care 50(4): 329–339
Charlton B 1996 All part of life's rich tapestry. Health Service Journal, 5 September: 16
Cupitt D 1988 The new Christian ethic. SCM, London
Hart J 1971 The inverse care law. Lancet 71: 495–503
Le Guin U 1988 In: Wilson M A coat of many colours. Epworth Press, London
Mahler H 1988 Address to World Health Assembly. In: Bellamy & Pyke, op cit
Maslow A 1970 Motivation and personality. Harper & Row, London
Moberg D 1979 Spiritual well being: sociological perspectives. University Press, Washington, DC
Moore W 1996 All stressed up and nowhere to go. Health Service Journal, 5 September: 22–24
Nouwen H 1972 The wounded healer. Doubleday, London
Pattison S 1991 Seeing justice done. Counselling 1991(3): 95–97
Pattison S 1994 Why we are not all disabled. Contact 113: 1
Pattison S 1995 Change not decay. Contact 116: 1
Pattison S 1997 The faith of the managers. Cassell, London
Priestley J 1996 Spirituality in the curriculum. Hockerill Educational Foundation, London.
Real World Coalition 1996 The politics of the real world. Earthscan, London
Rumbold B 1986 Helplessness and hope: pastoral care in terminal illness. SCM, London
Schumacher E 1974 Small is beautiful. Abacus, London
Wakefield G 1983 A dictionary of Christian spirituality. SPCK, London
Walter T 1985 All you love is need. SPCK, London
West M 1996 Mental health of the workforce in NHS trusts. In: Moore W, op cit.
Wilkinson R 1996 Unhealthy societies. Routledge, London

Index

Location references in bold indicate figures and tables